The
Healing Power
OF
ENERGIZED
WATER

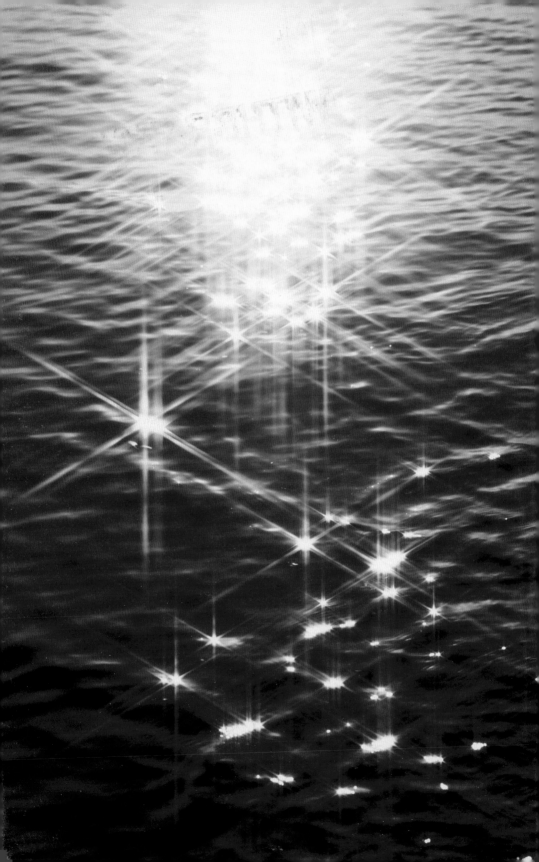

The
Healing Power
OF
ENERGIZED
WATER

**The New Science of Potentizing the
World's Most Vital Resource**

ULRICH HOLST

Translated by Jon E. Graham

Healing Arts Press
Rochester, Vermont • Toronto, Canada

Healing Arts Press
One Park Street
Rochester, Vermont 05767
www.HealingArtsPress.com

Healing Arts Press is a division of Inner Traditions International

Originally published in German under the title *Die Geheimnisse der Wasserbelebung* by Joy Verlag
First U.S. edition published in 2010 by Healing Arts Press

Note to the reader: *This book is intended as an informational guide. The remedies, approaches, and techniques described herein are meant to supplement, and not to be a substitute for, professional medical care or treatment. They should not be used to treat a serious ailment without prior consultation with a qualified health care professional.*

Library of Congress Cataloging-in-Publication Data
Holst, Ulrich.
  [Geheimnisse der Wasserbelebung. English]
  The healing power of energized water : the new science of potentizing the world's most vital resource / Ulrich Holst ; translated by Jon E. Graham. —1st U.S. ed.
      p. cm.
  Includes bibliographical references and index.
  ISBN 978-1-59477-338-9 (pbk.)
  1. Hydrotherapy. 2. Water. 3. Bioenergetics. I. Title.
  RZ999.H65 2004
  615.8'53—dc22

                                                                    2009046572
Printed and bound in India by Replika Press Pvt. Ltd.

10   9   8   7   6   5   4   3   2   1

Text design and layout by Virginia Scott Bowman
This book was typeset in Garamond Premier Pro and Frutiger with Garamond Premier Pro and Gill Sans as display typefaces

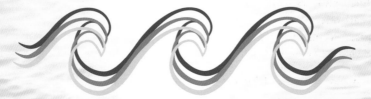

Contents

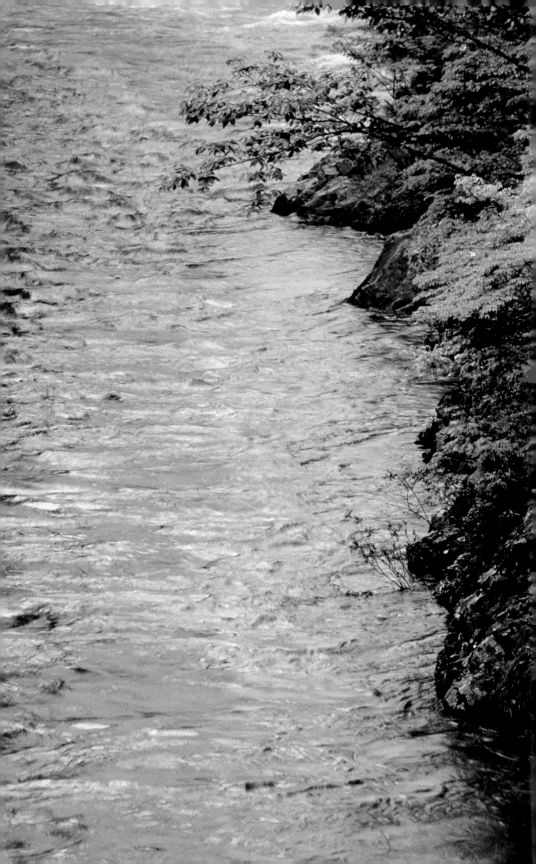

Acknowledgments

First, I would like to express my profound gratitude to water itself, just for existing. This book about water follows a trail blazed by many authors before me, who made my own task seem as easy and fluid as the element water.

Second, I would like to extend my gratitude to the many people involved in the dynamization of water. I had the good fortune to talk with many of them and all displayed the same cooperative spirit, even those who were commercial competitors. The element water seems to act like a bonding agent, offering itself as a meeting place where people can combine their strengths.

I would also, of course, like to thank all those who helped in the writing of this book. They helped transform an ordinary manuscript into something that is special in both content and appearance.

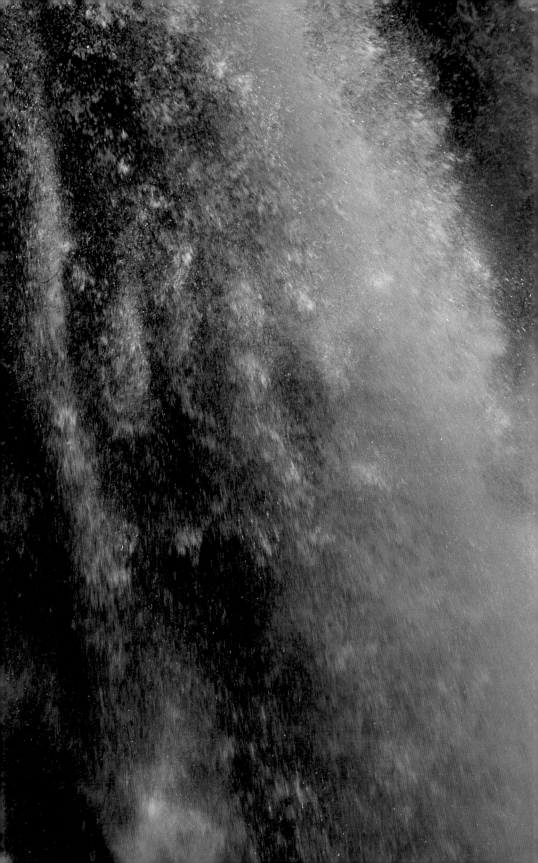

Introduction

A COUPLE OF YEARS ago while hiking in the Himalayan foothills of India, I had a somewhat unusual encounter with a young yogi meditating on a footbridge that spanned a raging torrent. He was sitting cross-legged, motionless as a statue, enveloped in a saffron yellow robe, with his long brown hair pulled back in a bun. His eyes were closed, and his meditation was so deep and intense that it seemed impossible for anything to disturb it. The sight of this ascetic literally stopped me in my tracks, and I just stared at him in total fascination for many minutes. At the time I conjectured that he'd most likely chosen this singular spot because it was a favorable environment for becoming entirely absorbed in his meditation. Indeed, the sound of running water is hypnotic. But today, after extensive study of the techniques and procedures for dynamizing water that has been contaminated or polluted, I now lean toward a second hypothesis: perhaps this yogi, in his many hours of meditation, was intending to transmit his noble spiritual vibrations into the water flowing several yards beneath his feet. In fact, this same water was essential to the survival of the inhabitants of entire towns and villages a few hundred miles farther downstream.

I will never know if this yogi really had the intention of vitalizing the water in the stream below him, or if the intention I loaned him was merely the product of my overactive imagination. I do know, however, that certain human beings, certain shapes, and certain stones or minerals have the power to confer amazing properties upon water, and even cure reputedly incurable diseases. This is why hundreds of thousands of pilgrims make their way to Lourdes in France every year, including many ill individuals searching for a cure; and why several million make the pilgrimage to every Kumbha-Mela festival in India to bathe in the polluted waters of the holy river. These waters somehow have a powerful capacity for triggering the body's natural ability to regenerate. Can the miracles and wonders allegedly conferred by certain waters be only the product of superstition? Are they merely vestiges of ancient beliefs?

The facts openly contradict this hypothesis. Recent scientific discoveries in the field of water studies make it possible to state unequivocally that water is not simply a banal liquid—nothing more than a chemical formula. Water is energy and the source of life. Water is endowed with memory and embodies a large quantity of very informative data. High-quality water is life giving and offers both energy and health, whereas heavily polluted or contaminated water can be the source of all kinds of illness and pathological disorders.

Ten years ago my wife and I decided to equip our house with a device for bioenergetically dynamizing our water. I have to admit that I was rather skeptical of all the amazing claims in the brochure that came with the appliance, but it kept all these promises, as well as others of which we had been completely unaware! Our tap water regained its flavor and lost most of its hardness. We could once again bathe without concern that the water would dehydrate our skin. Even our dog was delighted about this wonderfully regenerated water. He was now happy to drink what we gave him, whereas previously he preferred rain puddles to what came from our tap.

It was his reaction in particular that inspired me to study the element of water much more extensively and investigate the commercially available techniques for cleansing water, all of which have the potential to restore its potential as a vital energy.

At first my main questions were about polluted waters, especially heavily polluted waters. I wondered it they could be redynamized by means of these techniques. I also wondered if water could be conditioned without losing its innate, original qualities—and without the need to turn to a prophet like Elijah or an Indian yogi to get the job done right. The years I have spent researching this matter allow me to answer these questions in the affirmative.

I have written this book to give readers a multitude of options for resolving their individual issues with water. I've also suggested ways to use this essential element with more wisdom and discernment in everyday life. Although sensational, unfounded claims seem to be the rule, it is no exaggeration to say that without drinkable water, our very lives are at risk.

1

"Water Gives Life to All Things"

And he went forth unto the spring of the waters, and
cast the salt in there, and said, Thus saith the LORD,
I have healed these waters; there shall not be from
thence any more death or barren land.

2 KINGS 2:21

CLOSE TO CERTAIN WELLS that have been dug with great difficulty in the desert lands of Asia and Africa, it's common to see a sign proclaiming that "Water gives life to all things." People in lands that suffer dire water shortage have no illusions about its value—they know it is absolutely essential to their survival. There are two images that illustrate the crucial importance of this element in their lives: tufts of grass carving a path across the sands following torrential rains; and the harassed Bedouin carefully pulling a bucket of water from the depths of an oasis well to slake his thirst and that of his animals after long hours of walking through the desert under a beating sun. Rainwater nurtures the growth of blades of grass in the sand, and well water gives life and energy to the nomad and his herd. Not just the Bedouin, but all the inhabitants of the planet's desert regions have a profound respect and veneration for the element water. More than a mere liquid to satisfy thirst, cleanse the body and clothing, or sustain crops and fields, water is a sacred substance in their lives, worth far more than any treasure that could be amassed over a lifetime. This truth has been acknowledged by all the world's civilizations, as exemplified by these words inscribed on a boundary marker in the Kathmandu Valley of Nepal that was probably erected in the fourth century BCE:

> Everything has its origin in the element water.
> Everything will end in the element water.
> Everything has a vital need for water.
> May he who is without thirst refrain from wasting water!
> May he who is impure not neglect to honor water!

WATER SHAPES OUR WORLD

Water covers more than 70 percent of the globe. But what is the primordial origin of all these water masses? Has water always existed on our planet? Has our Earth always been the blue planet, as it now appears in photographs from space? Does Mars, too, have water, as it appears in images sent back by the 2004 space probe? We have no definitive answers to these questions, but perhaps the more inclusive question would be: Has water always existed in the cosmos? There are a number of clues that allow us to answer this question in the affirmative. For one, some space physicists report giant snowballs (seventy-five to eighty feet in diameter), or comets of ice, traveling regularly through the stratosphere in the direction of Earth, dispersing water as they are eroded by the solar wind. This phenomenon, it is said, goes back some 4.6 billion years. Could these be "rains of ice" emitted by outer space?

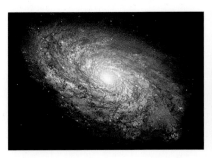
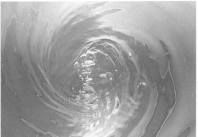

The launching of space probes opens new avenues for research but also raises new questions. Is water a primordial element, a constituent element of the universe and of the cosmos? Is the spiral the primordial form of all life? We encounter this form everywhere—in the outer galactic nebulae; in water, where it appears in a helix structure, a kind of winding spiral; and in DNA, whose very structure appears in the form of a double helix.

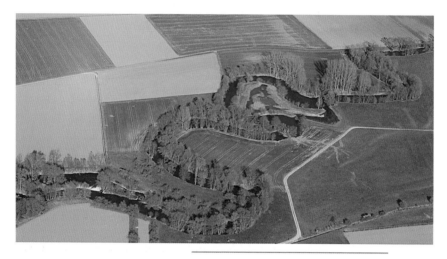

Winding or meandering lines are omnipresent in nature.

We need only look at nature (waterways, the trunk of an olive tree, conch shells, bones) and natural phenomena (typhoons, tornadoes) to realize that spiral movements, scrolling movements, meanderings, and snakelike winding movements are present everywhere in our world. Water shapes everything that exists in our vast cosmos, from the infinitesimally small to the infinitely large. Nature knows no right angles or straight lines. And, as illustrated on page 7, the Gulf Stream itself carves a sinuous path through the cold waters of the Atlantic.

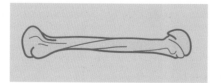

A spiral is clearly distinguishable on this bone.

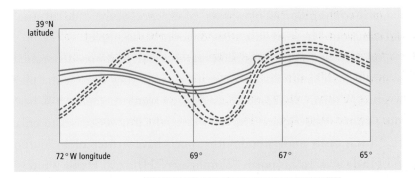

39°N
latitude

72° W longitude   69°   67°   65°

The Gulf Stream, a warm current in the Atlantic Ocean, follows a gigantic meandering course through much colder waters, a phenomenon that nature philosopher Theodor Schwenk explains in his book, *Sensitive Chaos: The Creation of Flowing Forms in Water and Air.**

FROM A BRIDGE OVER TROUBLED WATER TO WATER UNDER THE BRIDGE

There is no life without water. This is undoubtedly the reason why every language abounds in metaphors connected to water. We use all kinds of water-related expressions and rarely, if ever, ask ourselves about their origins. We talk about the "flow" of time, sports fans who "spill out" onto the streets from a stadium, someone who is a "river" of ideas, "streams" of gold (the profusion of rich decoration characteristic of Baroque churches), and a "flood" of responses. Even some terms from the realm of finance evoke the movement of water. For example, we read in business journals about an "inflow" of capital into the market, or that the stock exchange is "dropping" or "rising" like a river that is dwindling or threatening to flood its banks. A neighbor can be envied for "drowning" in wealth while our own fortunes are "running dry." The solution to a vexing problem is described as a "bridge over troubled waters," while "water under the bridge" refers to something that is past history. In the media journalists

*Publication information for this title as well as for other books referenced in the text is provided in Recommended Reading and Listening (page 143).

often refer to the outbreak of a "wave" of violence, or the "tide turning" in a bad situation. These are just a few of countless examples.

Our need and appreciation for water is our common denominator, recognized by all individuals, no matter where they live on the planet. The great William Shakespeare used many water metaphors. When he wrote, "Glory is like a circle in the water, which never ceases to enlarge itself," it was easily understood. Other poets have written of an "outpouring" of their love. In his poem "Tannhauser," Heinrich Heine wrote:

> *Ich liebe sie mit Allgewalt,*
> *Nichts kann die Liebe hemmen!*
> *Das ist wie ein wilder Wasserfall,*
> *Du kannst seine Fluten nicht dämmen;*
> *Er springt von Klippe zu Klippe herab,*
> *Mit lautem Tosen und Schäumen,*
> *Und bräch er tausendmal den Hals,*
> *Er wird im Laufe nicht säumen.*

> I love her, I love her with all my might,
> And nothing but my love can stay!
> 'Tis like a rushing waterfall,
> Whose force no man can sway;
> It dashes on from cliff to cliff,
> And roareth and foameth still.
> Though it breaks its neck a thousand times,
> Its course it would yet fulfill.

Love poems are saturated with water metaphors, many of which refer to the forms it takes in nature. This is hardly surprising, given the fact that the human body is comprised of 80 percent water. Furthermore, the ionic composition of blood plasma is nearly identical to that of seawater. Even the soul has been linked to water; the old Saxon word for soul was *saiwalo,* which can be approximately translated as "one who belongs to the sea," or "one whose origin is the sea." And it has been almost a century

since the term "depth psychology," which now has become an everyday expression, was first applied to psychoanalysis.

WATER AS MEDICINE

The famous German writer Goethe tells us "without water, there is no salvation,"* a reminder that water is essential and life supporting, and we forget this at our peril. Hippocrates, Paracelsus, Hildegarde of Bingen, and a number of famous healers and physicians throughout the centuries have recommended water as the first and best medicine. Drinking water before you become thirsty is a sensible precautionary approach for maintaining good health. Individuals drinking between two and three quarts (or approximately the same amount in liters) of pure water daily often rediscover the beneficial, and sometimes therapeutic, properties of water.

The human body requires a certain amount of water daily, without which it will be unable to properly perform its functions, because cellular fluids and the blood vessels stimulate the various metabolic systems. Lacking sufficient water, the cells and tissue become clogged and nutrients are no longer able to reach the vital organs.

The water we drink is not used equitably by all parts of the body. Medical science tells us, for example, that the brain's water needs are a priority (it's 78 percent water) and that as little as 2 percent insufficient water is enough to cause confused thinking and disorientation. This is why doctors and naturopaths recommend not waiting until you are thirsty to drink water. The body triggers the sensation of thirst when it is suffering a reduction in water reserves, and by then it may already be deficient by as much as 2 percent. For vitality and health, the human body needs from a quart and a half to two quarts of water every day. It would be extremely difficult to fulfill daily fluid requirements with liquids such as fruit juice, tea, and coffee. Although coffee and tea may help with hydration, the net percentage is far lower due to the caffeine they contain. This is one reason why coffee is served with a glass of water in some parts of the world.

Drinking adequate water on a daily basis will cause a certain num-

---

*From *Faust II*

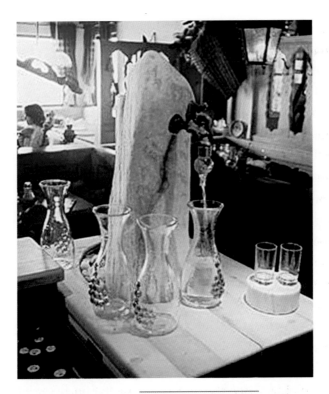

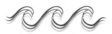
A water fountain made from a block of rock crystal that refines the quality of water

ber of disorders or physical ailments to vanish. Complaints ranging from backaches to ADD and asthma have reportedly been alleviated simply by increasing water consumption.

A BRIEF HISTORY OF BATHING

Bathing as an essential habit of good health dates all the way back to the Mesopotamian civilizations.

Baths in the Ancient East

In the land of the two rivers, the Tigris and the Euphrates, archaeologists have unearthed bathrooms in palaces dating from the second century BCE that were quite sophisticated for their era. In Mari, for example, near the border between Syria and Iraq, the royal family had an immense bathroom (236 square feet) equipped with two terra-cotta tubs. One evidently was used for cleansing the body, while the other was used for cosmetic and grooming purposes.

Warm baths have been long regarded as a factor in both physical and mental health. Bathing in hot water not only cleans out the pores but also loosens the muscles, calms the disposition, and restores zest for life.

Ancient Greece imitated the Eastern civilizations in the matter of baths, and we see this reflected in Homer's *Odyssey*. Upon his return to Ithaca, Ulysses was urged to take a hot bath, followed by a massage with precious oils—a custom native to the East.

But the Greek philosophers later felt compelled to claim that hot baths softened mind and body and called for the more Spartan discipline of cold water. Plato, for example, in his vision of the ideal city, *Politea*, recommends hot baths only for the ill and the elderly.

The Baths of Ancient Rome

Baths experienced expansive development in ancient Rome with the *thermae* (thermal baths). Vast and imposing, some thermae welcomed thousands of people every day. The thermae of Caracalla in Rome, inaugurated in 216 CE, had impressive dimensions: 680 feet long, 440 feet wide, and more than 100 feet high (beneath a dome). They could accommodate more than fifteen hundred bathers at a time. The ancient Roman baths had floor-based heating systems and offered a reading room, art gallery, and boutiques, as well as a variety of contemporary fitness techniques. The water required to run these establishments—approximately thirty thousand cubic feet a day—was piped in via a complex system of aqueducts.

The Roman aqueducts did an admirable job of supplying all the urban centers of the Roman Empire with potable water. Water was collected from springs reputed for their purity, then transported all the way into the cities (often 250 miles or farther). It is interesting to note that this system for transporting water clearly foresaw the need for twists and turns and included several stages where the water was swirled in whirlpools in order to preserve its natural regenerative capacities, purity, and

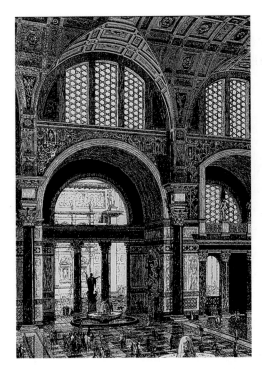

The Roman baths of Caracalla

original vitality. The engineers who designed this system obviously were trying to reproduce as closely as possible the natural conditions in which water circulates. This point is of major importance.

The Birth of Christianity Heralds a Decline in Bathing

In ancient Rome taking a bath was customary and common. But starting in the fourth century CE with Emperor Constantine—who signed the Edict of Milan introducing freedom of worship for Christianity—religious authorities began vilifying this beneficial practice and identifying public baths as quagmires for the soul and a source of carnal temptation. They warned their faithful to guard themselves against the dangers of bathing. In the fifth century Saint Augustine still tolerated a bath once a month, but Saint Jerome strongly counseled young girls against bathing unless it was in total darkness. This is a far cry from the God of Genesis, who, after each act of Creation, judged it good.

In the nineteenth century, Sebastien Kniepp, a German priest,

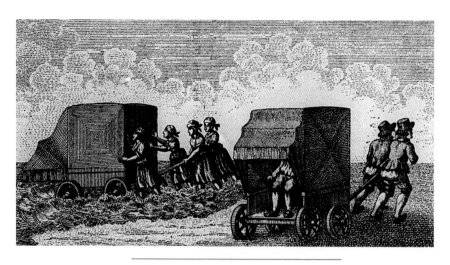

Bathing carts on Norderney Island (North Sea), around 1800

rediscovered the therapeutic properties of bathing. However, he did not go so far as to recommend hot baths but suggested cold water, which, as everyone knows, scarcely inspires any sensuousness.

THE WATER OF LIFE
CAN ALSO SOW DEATH

The year in which I began work on this book was one in which large parts of Europe were subjected to massive flooding. Austria, the Czech Republic, Italy, and Germany were all affected. The rains were so copious that they triggered landslides and brought considerable damage to both residential and agricultural areas. The catastrophe drove thousands of people from their homes. When the waters retreated, many people returned to find nothing but a field of ruins. Although it is the essence of life, the power of water can also cause destruction and death.

Fear of water is deeply anchored in the human mind. The collective unconscious appears never to have forgotten the stories of the great flood. The Old Testament recounts a deluge that carried off all of humanity except for Noah, his family, and pairs of animals; while Plato described a continent named Atlantis that had been swallowed by waves. In his possibly allegorical recounting, this catastrophe was the consequence of a comet striking the earth and triggering an instantaneous and dramatic rise in the water level. The sky was obscured by thick clouds of dust, which would have made atmospheric conditions unstable.

In our present world, it is the human lifestyle that is responsible for climate change and global warming. The melting polar ice caps could result in a substantial rise in sea levels, which could, in turn, trigger other disasters.

POTABLE WATER IS BECOMING SCARCE

The scarcity of potable water, a true tragedy, primarily affects the poor and underdeveloped parts of the world. This often forces the people of these lands to drink dirty water, which exposes them to all kinds of disease. A recent report issued by the World Health Organization in Geneva indicates some two hundred million individuals are currently affected by bilharziosis, a parasite-borne illness; and close to a billion people suffer from diarrhea-causing illnesses that result from drinking unclean water.

In many parts of the globe—including some Western countries—water has become a source of mortal danger. According to a study undertaken at the behest of President Bill Clinton while he was still in office, not one single river in the United States remains unsullied by chemical pollutants. After two centuries of industrialization, the "blood of the

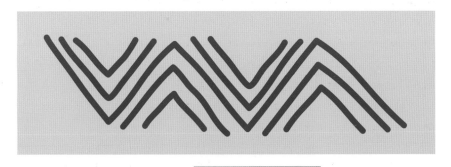

Representation of water by the Hopis

Earth Mother"—to borrow an expression dear to Native Americans—has suffered complete desecration.

In Austria recent studies reveal that half of the underground aquifers are polluted by nitrites and pesticides, and the situation in Germany, France, and Switzerland is equally dire. It is urgent that funds be allocated to cover the costs of cleansing these vital water sources. We have the technological means of cleaning soiled and polluted waters, even those that are heavily contaminated. Excellent results have been obtained using various commercial procedures, several of which will be examined in the following chapters of this book.

Pure water is becoming scarcer and more expensive across the planet. In the Western world we are consuming, on average, eight times more water than we were eighty years ago. In former times, potable water for a city like Munich or Chicago would have been provided, at least in part, by artesian wells. However, it takes an extremely long time (about ten thousand years) for these water sources to be replenished. In Western Europe water is recycled through an eight-stage treatment process. At the very minimum it requires the addition of chlorine, often followed by filtration and exposure to ultraviolet light, to make it potable again. Pure, life-giving water has become a rare commodity, even in Europe and North America. In these early years of the third millennium, we are on the eve of witnessing the fulfillment of what Austrian forester and visionary inventor Viktor Schauberger foresaw in 1935: "The time will come when a liter of water will cost as much as a liter of good wine."

2

The Peculiarities of Water

WATER BEHAVES IN A singular manner in comparison to the other elements, and sometimes its behavior can seem incomprehensible. To cite but one example, most natural substances become more dense when frozen. But water becomes less dense and weighs less at colder temperatures. This explains why the ice mass at the poles floats on the surface instead of sinking into the water, and ice cubes added to a glass of fruit juice or an alcoholic beverage immediately bob to the surface.

AN ENIGMA OF NATURE

If water behaved in accordance with the laws of nature, we would not be able to ice skate. In fact, it is the water from the bottom of ponds and rivers that begins to freeze, and not the water on the surface. Water reaches its maximum density and weight not at 32° Fahrenheit, but at 40° Fahrenheit. As it cools further it becomes less and less dense, and by the time it is completely crystallized (as ice) it is 9 percent less dense than water and will float to the surface. Thus warmer water is drawn toward the riverbed or pond bottom, providing a more consistent temperature for the inhabitants.

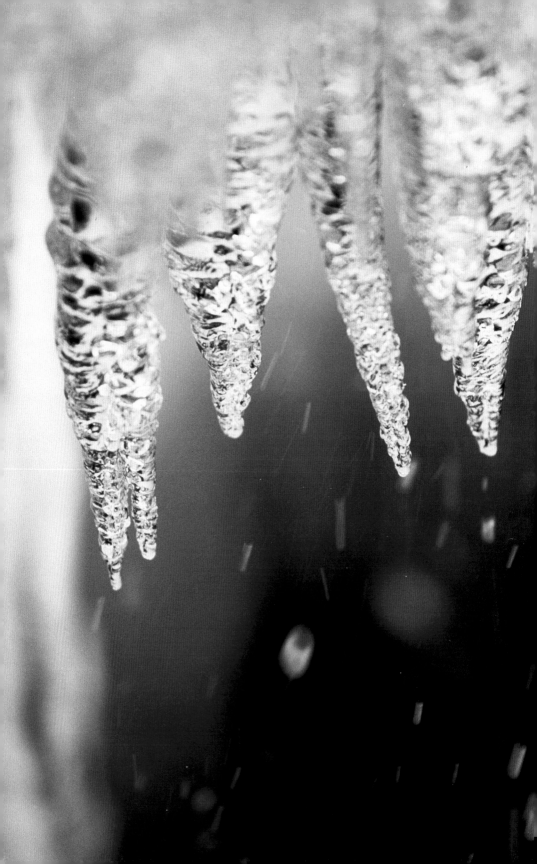

I can provide a second example of the unique behavior displayed by water: the constituent elements of water are oxygen and hydrogen, which are two gases, and yet water behaves like a liquid. This is because the molecules "stick together," or cluster, at moderate temperatures. At normal room temperature, there are about four hundred molecules combined to form one single, large molecule.

When water heats up, the bonds holding together the oxygen and hydrogen molecules become unstable, the number of molecules bound together diminishes, and water evaporates into the atmosphere as a gas. But water is a sociable substance and always seeks to bind with another fluid or substance. It is the preeminent example of a binding element. Researchers offer no clear explanation of this behavior.

Some scientists have developed a hypothesis for the human circulatory system based on the similarities between blood and water. They believe that because healthy blood, like fully developed water, is naturally ascendant, the heart doesn't pump blood through the arteries, but regulates circulation. A spring welling out of a rock is a clear illustration of water's ability to carve a path upward through the stone that would contain it.

Water: Creating a Bond between Earth and Sky

Rudolf Steiner and Theodor Schwenk, two nature philosophers with international reputations, interpreted water's unusual behavior in an unconventional way. What water shows by its unusual activities, they maintained, is that its original home is not planet Earth but the outermost reaches of the cosmos. Among the many clues that lend corroboration to their theory is water's natural tendency to ascend—from rock and up plant stems and tree trunks—defying the laws of gravity and terrestrial attraction to rise ever higher until it reaches the outer fringes of the atmosphere. Steiner and Schwenk explain this tendency of water as a phenomenon of memory. They believe that water holds the memory of its primordial home—the outer reaches of the cosmos.

This tendency of water makes it the element that creates a liaison between heaven and earth. It is no accident that water is present in so

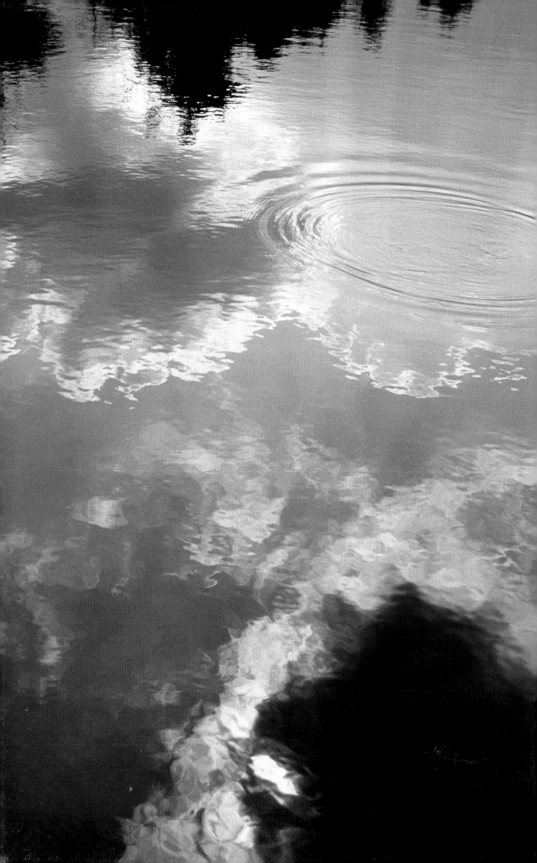

many spiritual ceremonies and rituals, such as the ritual baptisms of Christians and the daily ablutions of Hindus.

> *The human soul is like water*
> *From heaven it descends and to heaven it rises again;*
> *Then it must fall once more to earth,*
> *In eternal flux.*
>
> GOETHE

THE MEMORY OF WATER

If nature had no memory, there would be no evolution; all living things, including single-celled organisms, would always be forced to start over from nothingness. All living things, in whatever form they may appear—including the molecule and the atom—cannot help but be endowed with memory and must pass on the fruits of their experience. Otherwise, there would be nothing but stagnation.

Memory's capacity is closely linked to DNA and has the structure of DNA—a double spiral or double helix—a pattern that cannot help but bring to mind the double spirals in the movement of water: a spiral coiling to the right and a spiral coiling to the left. Is this also water's power of recall?

Water molecules are continuously attracting one another, like magnets. Water is in constant flux; its quality changes from one instant to the next as a consequence of the number of combined molecules, the ways in which they are combining, and so forth. This explains why no two flakes of snow or two drops of water are ever truly identical. Some people may find this difficult to believe, but it is the reality.

Clusters of molecules are always unique. They can be compared, to a certain extent, to human beings: the nature of a group of people depends upon the state of mind of those in the group. People who have gathered to enjoy an outdoor concert are in a different state of mind from those who have assembled for a street demonstration, but seen from a distance they are difficult to differentiate, especially if the groups are almost identical in size.

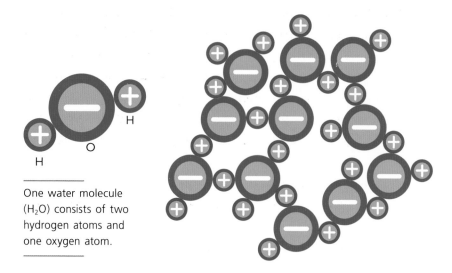

One water molecule (H$_2$O) consists of two hydrogen atoms and one oxygen atom.

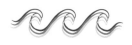

Because of their magnetic charge, water molecules attract one another to form a group of molecules, a phenomenon more properly described as a "cluster." Clusters continually form and break apart, depending on what external influences they are subject to, as well as what is molding them internally.

Anyone who operates from the principle that water is only ever water, and believes the formula H$_2$O is its entire identity, is comparable in some ways to a viticulturist who is satisfied by simply slapping a "wine" label on all the bottles from one harvest, no matter what their different grape varieties. In other words, this is not someone who appreciates differences in quality.

Water's Lasting Impressions

A person who takes part in a demonstration is subject to a number of impressions, and these impressions don't dissipate when the demonstrators disperse at the end of the event. The same principle can be applied to water. To make it easier to grasp the phenomenon of water memory, imagine water in a swimming pool. The quality of the water in a pool changes throughout the day. In the early morning the water in a swimming pool has a different quality from the evening water that has been used all day long. The morning pool water tends to communicate a sense of calm and balance to the swimmer, whereas by the end of the afternoon the pool water is likely to convey agitation and nervousness. The reason for this difference is that all the people who used the pool that day have passed their own imprints and electrical energy into the water. Stress collected by swimmers at their workplaces or elsewhere affects the quality of the water. These stress imprints are usually perceived indirectly, and swimmers respond with more or less feverish or disorganized movements of their arms or legs. Water retains the memory of all the impressions it receives, both the good and the bad. In the evening, even if only one person remains in the pool, that swimmer runs a strong risk of absorbing at least some of the many various impressions with which the water was charged over the day.

In the same way, even filtered water can retain the memory of pesticides and other poisons that are routinely released into the atmosphere or spread on lawns and fields. For this reason, more and more people have totally stopped drinking tap water. (Statistics show that the annual consumption of mineral water went from twelve and a half liters [thirteen quarts] per person in 1970 to one hundred fifteen liters [more than thirty gallons] per person in 2003. In other words, it grew more than tenfold in thirty-three years.)

Many studies have been conducted in an attempt to discover the actual duration of water's memory, but none to this point have been comprehensive enough. Some influencing factors appear to dissolve after only a few minutes, whereas others seem to persist for several days or months. Water's memory is somewhat comparable to that of human beings: we quickly forget the minor annoyances but feel the impact of serious traumas for a long time, if not our entire lives.

The atomic and subatomic memory of water is no fabrication; it absolutely, purely exists. The proof of this can be found in the action of highly diluted homeopathic medications. Microscopes, no matter how powerful, are unable to detect the slightest trace of the initial substance—arsenic, for example—in these dilutions. From a biochemical perspective, the water of a highly diluted homeopathic medicine has no distinctive characteristics.

However, this does not prevent the water from retaining its memory of the initial substance. Skeptics may continue to posit the placebo effect of these medications, but what can they say when an animal or plant recovers its energy and vigor as a result of homeopathic treatment? There is no proven argument that animals and plants are susceptible to the power of self-suggestion!

Water is unquestionably endowed with memory. So, if we turn our minds for a moment to all the noxious substances that are constantly spilling into our water supplies, there is plenty of reason to be nervous.

There are many things poisoning our "well." Consider the runoff from industrial feed for factory farms, as well as the animal waste and slaughter by-products that accumulate in the water waste and often go into porous septic systems. In high-yield agriculture, vegetables and grains are treated with a whole range of chemical products, some of which are extremely harmful to the earth, air, and water supply. When genetically modified fruits and vegetables are exposed to radiation to prolong their shelf life, this, too, passes into the earth's systems both directly and indirectly—through our bodily wastes. Industry is notorious for carelessly dumping vast amounts of liquid wastes directly into nearby oceans and rivers. All of these things are saturated to some extent by the mental states and emotions of the people involved in their production. And all have a subtle effect on the consumer.

On the positive side, it has been noted many times that any food or drink prepared with love always has more flavor.

Positive or negative, the past continues to vibrate in everything in the form of micro-information. Although no device yet exists capable of detecting it on the biophysical plane, we know this to be true.

Water's Memory Made Visible

We may not be able to measure it, but the micro-information contained in water has been photographed. During the 1960s, anthroposophist and water specialist Theodor Schwenk took photographs of water drops that are quite remarkable.

More recently, Japanese doctor Masaru Emoto, an avid researcher of water, published several books of his photos of water crystals, which have enjoyed wide circulation. His images are as amazing as those taken by Schwenk.

Masaru Emoto: Water Crystal Photos

The procedure used by Masaru Emoto consisted of refrigerating water drops then photographing the crystals that formed in the cooling process. He has studied water from hundreds of different sources, including rivers, lakes, tap water, and sacred sites. The discoveries he has gleaned from them are truly thought provoking.

Readers will not be surprised to learn that pure water crystals have a beautiful hexagonal structure, whereas crystals formed by polluted water, or those that have been subjected to intense stress, are either incomplete or have irregular molecular clusters. The morphology of a water crystal can also change as a result of sound vibrations, or even by being in close proximity to words or phrases written on a piece of paper. The energetic waves emitted in meditation generally have a harmonizing effect on water crystals in the vicinity. There are multiple examples of this phenomenon in nature.

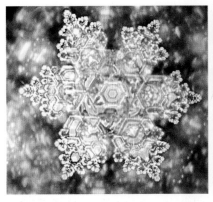 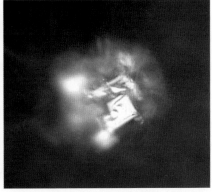

Water crystal from Saijo—a Japanese spring (*The Hidden Messages in Water*, by Masaru Emoto)

Water crystal from Dresden tap water (*The Hidden Messages in Water*, by Masaru Emoto)

The Hagalis Method

The Hagalis method of distillation, devised by German researcher and healer Andreas Schulz, reveals the unique micro-information contained in a specific water sample, or cluster of water molecules. A number of manufacturers of water revitalization appliances find the Hagalis method useful for illustrating the effectiveness of their equipment to potential customers and other interested parties.

The first stage of the Hagalis method consists of distilling the water. The residues are then mixed with ashes and calcium until they form crystals, which are then combined with the distilled liquid and painted over a laboratory slide. At this stage the water is allowed to vaporize at room temperature, which allows very clear contours and shapes to be revealed. They can be closely examined when enlarged under a microscope.

You'll find more crystalline water images at the inventor's website,

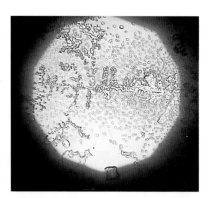

Crystals from Zurich: nonrevitalized tap water (enlarged four hundred times)

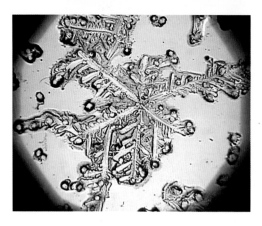

Crystals of the same water after it has been revitalized using bioenergetic methods (enlarged four hundred times). This photo is in stark contrast to the previous one in its clear definition of crystals. Here the crystals show sixty-degree angles, which indicates beneficial water quality. The presence of ninety-degree angles indicates low-quality water.

www.hagalis.de. The same site describes other crystal categories that are equally interesting, including those in food products, tissue from diseased organs, and so on.

Manufacturing a Magnificent Water Crystal

Anyone can learn how to distinguish ordinary tap water from that same water that has been revitalized. You'll need ice cubes of the water you wish to study, so be sure to make those before starting your project. Have the following tools and materials on hand when you begin:

- ⇜ A freezer unit
- ⇜ Ice cubes made from the water you intend to analyze
- ⇜ A glass or ceramic casserole dish with a lid
- ⇜ A roll of aluminum foil
- ⇜ Very thin cotton string (avoid synthetic fibers)
- ⇜ A thin piece of wood (for example, a wooden match with the sulfur tip removed)
- ⇜ At least one pint of the water you wish to study (in liquid form)
- ⇜ A magnifying glass (or camera with a zoom lens)
- ⇜ Fabric tape

Once you have your tools assembled, you can begin to manufacture your first water crystal. Be sure to have a sufficient supply of ice from the water you're analyzing, enough to half-fill the casserole dish.

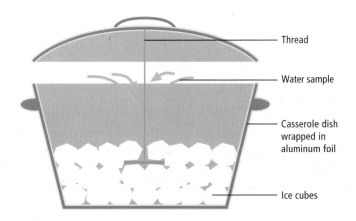

Thread

Water sample

Casserole dish wrapped in aluminum foil

Ice cubes

Before pouring the ice cubes into the casserole, cover the inside or the outside of the casserole dish and lid in aluminum foil to prevent the ice cubes from absorbing any electromagnetic rays coming from the immediate surroundings. Next, cut a piece of string (it should be long enough to go deep into the dish and almost touch the bottom); affix one end of the string to the bottom of the lid with a strip of cloth tape. Carefully rinse the ice cubes with the same water you are analyzing so they are free of any residual micro-information from a different water. Now you can pour the ice cubes into the casserole (which, remember, should fill it halfway) and place it in your freezer or the freezer compartment of your refrigerator. Adjust the temperature to its coldest setting.

When you think the casserole has been inside the freezer long enough to get sufficiently cold, take it out, remove the lid, and very carefully pour a little less than one-fourth cup of water over the string. Immediately replace the lid on the casserole dish and put it back into the freezer. Let it remain there for at least one and a half hours. Then very carefully remove it from the freezer. Slowly and gently raise the lid, taking care to keep it perfectly vertical. The now-frozen string will detach from the lid and remain vertical (see adjacent illustrations). With a little luck, you will see a superb ice crystal around the string. If this is the case, photograph it immediately or study it under a magnifying glass, because it will inevitably melt quite quickly.

A crystal like the one you see in the photo will most likely not be obtained on the first try. You may have to be quite persistent—one might say stubborn—to get one of this quality. Masuro Emoto himself, as he tells us in his books, sometimes had to perform this operation fifty times before obtaining a crystal worth photographing.

Bioenergetically Revitalizing Water
Using Water's Sensitivity

In the final analysis, water's extreme sensitivity and reactive power is an advantage. It implies that shapeless clusters of water are easy to break down, indicating that it is just as easy to prompt water of varying quality to restructure itself in a more harmonious form.

This is the fundamental notion that underlies all the methods for

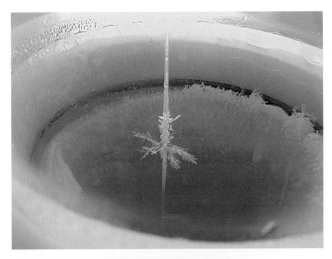

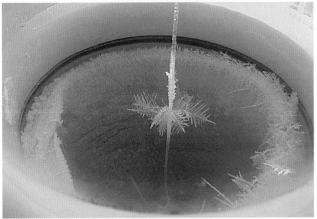

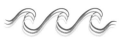

Tap water from Lucerne, Switzerland. The water in the top photo has not been treated, whereas the water in the bottom photo has been bioenergetically revitalized.

revitalizing water bioenergetically. Various procedures or techniques allow impulses to be communicated to tainted or polluted water that will erase any previously established undesirable programming and restore its original vitality. (The photos of ice crystals lend support to this theory of healthy transformation.)

Given the microscopic size of a water molecule, it goes without saying that the impulses used should be quite subtle (and their existence alone is sufficient to trigger these positive effects). A single glass of water contains billions of water molecules, more than half of which are in the process of restructuring, which is why water droplets and puddles form whenever water is poured on a flat surface.

Before getting into the core subject of this book—the various procedures for the revitalization of water and the inventors who devised them—I am going to briefly describe the principal categories of water and the characteristics of each category. This information is essential for evaluating the quality of a given kind of water and whether it requires revitalization.

THE DIFFERENT CATEGORIES OF WATER AND THEIR PRIMARY USES

Juvenile Water

Juvenile water is a geological term that means the water in question has not yet attained its maturity. To be more precise, this water is poor in trace elements and mineral salts. Juvenile water flows deep in the bowels of the earth and is often released as the steam accompanying volcanic eruptions. If we drank nothing but juvenile water, the trace elements and salts naturally present in our bodies would be depleted rapidly because this water would appropriate them and eventually be eliminated with it from the body as waste products. Our nails, teeth, bones, and hair would crumble and break.

Water that has naturally attained maturity by rising to the earth's surface at its own pace and emerging in the form of a spring has had ample time to become enriched with mineral salts. It has had the time, one might say, to acquire "experience." Water of this kind provides life for all living things: humans, animals, and plants.

A water that is brought to the surface artificially—for example, by drilling and piping it from the water table—is in no way close to maturity. This explains why the majority of tap water remains semi-juvenile. Water of this nature could remove more mineral salts and trace elements from the human body than it provides, thus depleting the energy of the person drinking it. Thus, someone can easily drink between two or three quarts of water a day—a more than sufficient quantity—without enjoying any of the presumed benefits. To compensate for the deficiencies in mineral salts and trace elements in some tap water, manufacturers of water activation and vitalization devices have anticipated the need to process the tap water through a layer of carefully selected stones and minerals. Other water revitalization devices are equipped with a system that provides readings on mineral content (this information will be provided later in the book, along with descriptions of the benefits offered by these devices).

Juvenile water is not suitable for drinking but is fine for washing. The same is true for rainwater, as I'll explain below.

Mature Water

Mature water from a mountain spring contains the appropriate proportions of carbon and mineral salts. It has been fully vitalized and energized by the movement it was long subjected to in the bowels of the earth. Fully mature water may not look much different from other water, but it has had many years to develop its life-giving properties. A mature water is crystal clear and has a slightly bluish tinge.

Bottling water under pressure diminishes its quality. If the bottles are made of plastic, the water will be stripped yet further of its original cargo of micro-information. Plastic materials have their own "memory," and plastic bottles are often manufactured with bisphenol A (BPA), which has been linked to diabetes and cardiovascular disease. A study supported by Harvard University showed that just one week of drinking cold liquids from a polycarbonate bottle increased BPA by more than two-thirds. Glass is preferred for its neutral vibrations and nontoxic composition.

Mineral Waters

As I mentioned earlier in the book, the consumption of mineral water has multiplied tenfold over the past several decades, largely in response to the slow but constant deterioration in tap water quality. Mineral waters have attained maturity since they originate, by definition, from springs that

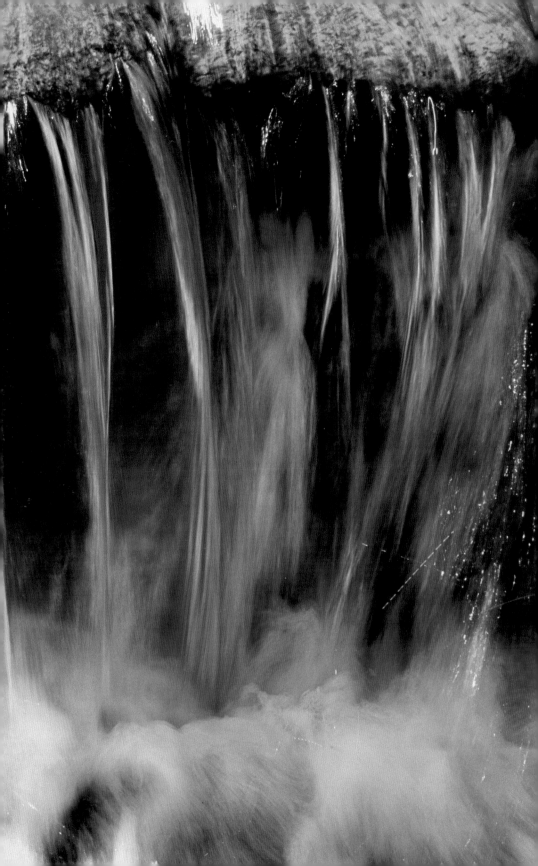

contain a certain minimum level of mineral salts. Sometimes carbon dioxide is added to mineral water to make it carbonated and perhaps intensify its flavor. The name "mineral water" implies that the water contains at least one gram of mineral substances, such as iron, potassium, and magnesium.

Ecologists are opposed to bottling water. In addition to the waste caused by manufacturing plastic bottles, many of them are not recycled but sent to the dump, and transporting bottles to consumers also creates pollution. As for the medical establishment, doctors and naturopaths alike cast a skeptical eye on the consumption of carbonated mineral water because it is acidifying and disturbs the healthy acid-alkaline balance of the body. Furthermore, the human body is not capable of ingesting all mineral salts, so there is an additional burden imposed on the organs responsible for the elimination of wastes.

Physicians generally recommend that their patients drink natural spring water, one that has not been subjected to any chemical treatment. As we shall see, people also have the option of drinking "revitalized water." Water of this nature offers three advantages: it preserves natural water reservoirs, avoids the filling of bottles under pressure, and eliminates the need for transporting bottles.

Well Water

Some people still have the good fortune of experiencing natural springs that freely dispense water to all who desire to drink. For example, Mt. Shasta City in northern California has a spring water fountain on a corner of the town's main street. Before modern technology, the drilling of a well was a complicated and risky undertaking, especially in the absence of water at the surface. In those days it was necessary to detect the place where the underground water source flowed closest to the surface. This was the job of the water witch, or the "water smeller" (a term commonly used in Switzerland), or water diviner. So essential was the local well that anyone who poisoned its water would be sentenced to death.

In Western Europe, where there is an abundance of water, it isn't difficult to find a water vein and dig a well. For water used in gardening or to quench the thirst of farm animals, some wells filter water through a layer of gravel. The procedure consists of arranging a fine layer of gravel between the filter pipe and the saturated soil, which prevents the pipe from becoming clogged by sand or mud.

The quality of water from a well or natural spring obviously depends upon its source—either a water vein or an aquifer. Natural mountain spring water is generally of excellent quality. In the plains, however, it almost always comes from the upper layers of the water table, which increasingly are tainted, mainly by liquid manure, or polluted by poisons used in factory farming and high-yield agriculture.

Rainwater

Rainwater is considered to be a juvenile water because evaporation has caused the loss of much of its mineral salt content. Furthermore, it absorbs all kinds of industrial wastes that are suspended in the atmosphere. These wastes are the cause of "acid rain," which, as we all know, poses a health threat to all living things: trees, plants, animals, and human beings.

It isn't advisable to drink rainwater, even when it is of good quality, and anyone who makes a regular habit of drinking melted snow will eventually begin to suffer from serious deficiencies. Like juvenile water, rainwater and melted snow steal the trace elements and mineral salts naturally present in the body, which are then eliminated in bodily waste.

As I mentioned earlier, clean rainwater is just fine for washing laundry. Not only will it get clothes clean, but it is also a natural softener. Acid rain water is not only unsuitable for drinking but also is not good for laundry. It is barely acceptable for watering the lawn and flowerbeds and not advisable for watering fruit trees or vegetable gardens. The toxins contained in acid rain will soon find their way into our digestive tracts.

Surface Waters

All water contains mineral salts and trace elements, and their quantity depends upon their source: springs, underground wells, rainwater, and so forth. It is increasingly common for these different waters to also contain undesirable substances: chemical residue from industry or agriculture and acid rain from the atmosphere.

Water from the surface is affected by daylight and a certain amount of sunlight, the intensity of which varies according to location and time of the year. Because water is a cold element by nature, it prefers shadowy regions and chill air. Heat causes it to lose oxygen, which has a tendency to make it tasteless. In addition, water that has too much exposure to the sun is more readily subject to the growth of bacteria and algae.

Tap Water

Humankind has always sought ways to have water on demand, which is completely understandable. Earlier cultures created goatskin flasks and designed pitchers for convenient transport and storage of water. People have captured it from springs and forced it into irrigation ditches for their crops. They have constructed canals and built series of pipes and water mains to bring it into their cities. Today, we have very sophisticated networks for water distribution at our disposal, but the water is of inferior quality.

Providing the upper floors of an apartment building with water

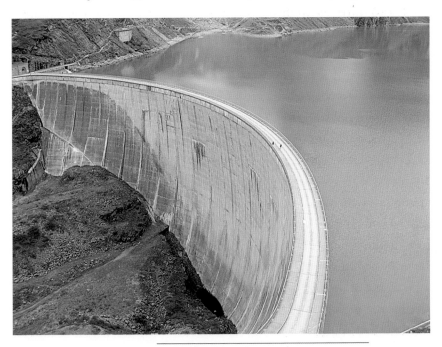

Dams contribute greatly to our ability to provide water on demand.

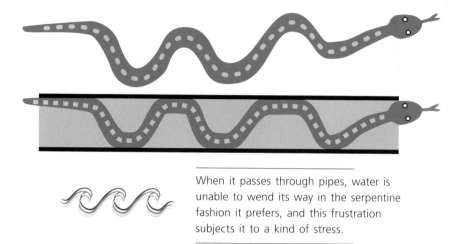

When it passes through pipes, water is unable to wend its way in the serpentine fashion it prefers, and this frustration subjects it to a kind of stress.

requires subjecting the water to high pressure. This process causes great stress to the water, which is reflected in its molecular groupings, or clusters. The reactive power of water like this is diminished, meaning it is less able to dissolve or absorb other substances. To get laundry or dishes clean with water of such mediocre quality, you'll need to use much more laundry powder or dishwashing liquid than you would need with clean rainwater or revitalized water. (Stressed tap water does offer one advantage over water that is not stressed: it doesn't absorb as much copper, lead, or other undesirable substances.) The hardness that is characteristic of stressed water has nothing in common with a water's "degree of hardness," which pertains to amounts of minerals in the water.

The molecule clusters in water that have been compressed under stress are harmful to your health. Regularly drinking polluted tap water will engender physiological disorders that, in turn, can cause difficulty dissolving and eliminating impurities. These impurities will then be stored in your joints and on the walls of your blood vessels. Over time this could result in a grating sound when you turn your head to the right or left, as if sand had been deposited between your cervical vertebrae. The insufficient elimination of impurities from the body may also cause deposits and calcifications that could someday cause a blood clot (thrombosis).

Water that is pressurized is also less able to supply the body (the cells) with the essential substances needed to maintain well-being: proteins and enzymes perform their duties much more effectively if the physiological fluids are flowing freely and not obstructed by molecular compaction.

Tap water may quite easily conform to current biochemical standards and even be pleasant tasting yet still have molecular consolidation, making it difficult to dispense energy and health to the person drinking it. You may recall the extreme sensitivity of water that was discussed at the beginning of this chapter. For example, it has been shown quite explicitly that even when tap water no longer shows any residue of prescription medication on the molecular level, it may continue to be permeated with the memory of that substance.

Drinking naturally healthy and sound water, or water that has been restored to that state by a revitalization process, rather than polluted tap water, will undoubtedly cause some physical disorders to vanish, or at least diminish. As we shall see later, revitalization procedures are capable of ridding polluted waters of their molecular compaction, as well as the memory of the undesirable substances resulting from such pollution.

Boiled Water

To make polluted or dirty water healthy, it can be boiled—a procedure as old as the world. Boiling tainted water not only kills germs and bacteria but also weakens and dissolves the memory these germs and bacteria have generated. Boiled water is also better at absorbing the active principles in tea leaves or plants used to prepare herbal brews and, of course, cleans laundry more efficiently.

The dissolution of the information contained in water molecules depends upon the length of time the water is boiled; brief boiling for just a few seconds will allow it to lose its memory only briefly. As the water cools down, there is a strong risk it will reconstruct itself.

Ayurvedic medicine, the traditional healing modality of India, recommends that water be boiled for seven minutes. Drinking this water while it is still lukewarm reinforces the body's natural capabilities of purification and detoxification. Several minutes of boiling appears to greatly improve water's ability to dissolve and transport.

Chinese medicine concurs with Ayurvedic medicine on this point.

According to Chinese practitioners, a long boiling period revitalizes water, which is beneficial for health. Drinking cold water, however, robs energy from the digestive organs, an energy they need in order to perform their functions properly. This is why the Asian custom is to serve hot water rather than cold beverages with meals. Hot water is the most common drink across the entire Asian continent.

Distilled Water

Distilled water is commonly used for refrigeration systems, steam pressing, in car batteries, and in sterilization of medical and food products. Distillation consists of bringing water to a boil until it begins to vaporize, leaving mineral sediment behind. The vapor is collected in a container, and once it cools again, it turns back into liquid.

Distilled water has lost a large part of its molecular memory to such an extent that it cannot support other substances. Bacteria have a very difficult time surviving in distilled water, and mineral substances are lost on contact with steam. There is, therefore, no sediment. Distilled water has no nutritive value and therefore provides no energy to the person drinking it. Its quality is very similar to clear or juvenile water.

Revitalizing distilled water with bioenergetic techniques is no easy task. It can only be dynamized and reactivated through contact with non-distilled water.

Morning Dew

Morning dew is condensed humidity. Its molecular structure is subtle and almost ethereal, and its therapeutic properties are renowned.

Some healing spas advocate taking early morning walks when the grass is still damp with dew. We should not overlook this ancient tradition as a technique for strengthening the body. Walking in the early morning enlivens body, mind, and soul. It allows us to capture the very distinctive vibrations of the dawn and the new day, as well as the fine "celestial rain" that mists over the earth's surface at night. Indeed, the Bible compares the gifts of the Holy Spirit to the "celestial dew" that fills the wilted soul with rays of divine light.

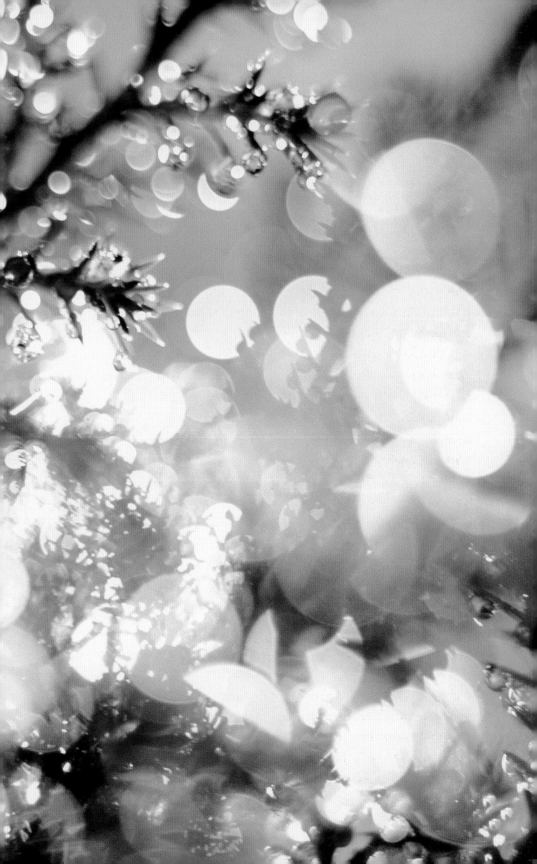

WATER CATEGORIES AND THEIR CHARACTERISTICS

Categories of Water \ Characteristics	Structure of the Water Molecules	Mineral Content
Semi-juvenile Water (well water drawn from the earth)	Structure is rarely complex	Very little (robs the body of minerals)
Mature Water	Harmonious and complex structure	Balanced (provides the body with valuable mineral salts)
Mineral Water	Harmonious and complex structure; molecular compaction once it has been bottled	Contains more mineral salts than the body needs (can cause metabolic overload)
Natural Spring Water	Varies from one water source to another but also depends on construction of the well	Varies from one source of water to the next
Rainwater, Snowmelt	Little complexity in structure; molecular compaction, depending upon pollution in the atmosphere	Little content (robs the body of its minerals)
Surface Water	Disharmonious structure and molecular compaction, depending upon the degree of air and soil pollution	Depends upon the composition: spring water, rainwater, or water from an underground water table, or aquifer
Tap Water	Inharmonious structure; molecular compaction, depending upon the origin of the water and the plumbing system	Depends upon the water's degree of hardness; forms deposits as a result of molecular compaction
Boiled Water (minimum seven minutes)	Complexity depends upon the water's origin; molecular compaction is almost nonexistent (and has a fragile structure if present)	Is a result of the water's origin
Distilled Water	Not very complex; chaotic structure	Does not contain any significant amount
Water Revitalized Using Dynamization Techniques	Harmonious and complex structure	Does not contain any, but certain devices imprint mineral information or pass the water directly through a mineral solution, thus increasing mineral content

Pollution from Sludge, Silt, or Pollutants; Remembers Pollutants	Pollution Resulting from Pressurization (and other factors)	Ability to Bind and Transport Properties (sediment, slag, food products, enzymes, cement, paint, and so on)	Cleaning Ability
None (potential contamination by contact with polluted underground waters)	Pump pressure	Good	Good
None (potential contamination by contact with polluted underground waters)	Not under pressure unless it is bottled	Excellent	Excellent
None (potential contamination by contact with polluted underground waters)	Pressure almost always induced at the time it is pumped, travels through water pipes, or is bottled; is enriched with CO_2	Weak, but only in the event of high mineral content	(Not applicable)
Is dependent upon the quality of the water source and the well's filtering system	Any pressure is the result of the well's pump system	Dependent upon the quality of the water source and well construction	Dependent upon the quality of the water source and the well construction
Is dependent upon the degree of atmospheric pollution	No pressure	Good	Good (as long as the water is pure)
Is dependent upon the degree of air and soil pollution	Pressure potentially induced at time it is pumped	Average	Unsuitable
Depends upon regulations enforced by current legislation; the memory is retained	Excessive pressure as a result of pumping and traveling through pipes	Weak	Rather poor, but dependent upon the degree of purity of the water
Is dependent upon the water's origins; the memory is almost wiped clean	Stress due to pumping is almost entirely eliminated	Excellent	Excellent
None, in principle	Stress due to pumping is almost entirely eliminated	Weak	Basically unsuitable
Organic substances: minimized; Nonorganic substances: minimized under certain conditions; memory neutralized	Stress as a result of pumping is minimized; oxygen deficiencies are balanced	Yes (substances remain suspended in the water)	Excellent

Consecrated Water

Water is regarded as sacred by all the world's great religions and is an essential part of numerous rituals and ceremonies. In Christianity water is an essential element of the sacrament of baptism (through which a newborn or convert is accepted into the religion), and the faithful bless themselves with holy water at the entrance to the church. Throughout the world priests and shamans are called to bless new buildings—homes, stables, paddocks, stores, and so forth—with holy water.

Do these consecration rituals necessarily fall under the heading of superstition? Not at all. In fact, consecrating water transmits a message of a sacred nature. As we have already seen, water is very sensitive to vibrations, and the message with which this water is charged at the time of consecration will be passed along to the next "user" of the water or of the consecrated building.

Helen Schulz, a certified therapist, told me of a very interesting experience she had, which I reproduce here with her consent.

I frequently give courses and seminars at a large swimming pool on the roof of a modern apartment building in Freiburg, which is on the western edge of the Black Forest region in Germany. It contains the standard level of chlorine and has been heated to 95° Fahrenheit expressly for us. During a recent weekend I gave a Watsu* workshop where we had complete freedom to experiment with percussion instruments, sing, and recite mantras.

Every night, we took samples of this water—one of the participants was an energy therapist—because we wanted to see its subsequent kinesiological energy. At the end of each day of Watsu, energy work, songs, and vibrations created by the percussion instruments, the quality of the water of the pool turned out to be significantly better than at the beginning of the day. On the following Monday the water was subjected to routine official inspection, and its quality was judged excellent. But there was one surprising thing—the analysis showed the water was of many times improved quality but

---

*Information about the healing modality of Watsu is available at the following websites: http://watsu.com, http://waba.edu, and www.watsu.org.nz.

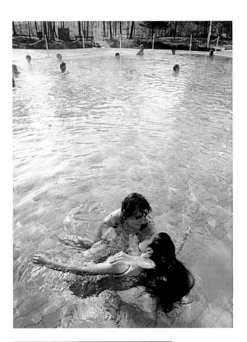

A Watsu session in a swimming pool in
Freiburg, Germany

had an abnormally low chlorine level, although the chemical had
been automatically added to the pool water every day.

The inspector was unable to explain this phenomenon. The
owner of the swimming pool was delighted, since the improved
quality allowed her to cut back on chlorine. For me, the results of
the analysis were not truly so surprising. The bodywork that took
place in these aquatic surroundings consisted of harmonious movements, and movements of this nature could not help but change the
vibrational quality of the water. Additionally relevant was the state
of mind of the participants during the sessions: the feelings of sym-
pathy that moved them, their tender ministrations to each other during the Watsu treatment, and the reverberations on the water of the
sacred sounds of the mantras and of the percussion instruments.

The Watsu sessions consequently had a dual effect: the healing of
the participants and the healing of the water via the participants.

The biophysical changes in the water quality in this swimming pool were really astonishing. The chlorine seemed to have partially vanished into thin air, by some kind of magic. Some may find this impossible to believe, because it contradicts the most elementary laws of chemistry. We will revisit this point in a later chapter.

For the moment, I advise the reader to closely study the water crystals reproduced in Masuru Emoto's books, particularly the photographs of water crystals taken from sacred sites, in this instance, Shinto and Buddhist temples in Japan. These water crystals are little short of miraculous, both for the beauty of their shapes and their harmonious structure. It would seem to confirm that the quality of holy waters is actually superior to that of ordinary water.

Before ending this chapter, I would like to cite several examples of rituals in different religious cultures that involve the element water. In Mexico, for example, the midwife at the birth of a child prays while washing the baby's tiny body and asks God to spare the child from illness and other calamities that caused his parents to suffer. The faithful who visit any of the Shinto sanctuaries at Ise Bay in Japan wash their feet in the Isuzu River, then rinse their mouths with this same water. The Bedouins of the Sinai sprinkle themselves with water before each prayer.

We have now reached the end of chapter 2, the main purpose of which was to introduce the different characteristics and properties of healthy water that is a true provider of life. The reader may now begin to grasp that an amazing reality is hidden behind the banal chemical formula of H_2O. The reader will also comprehend by now how much our survival depends on good-quality water that regenerates both mind and body. Water is simultaneously a beverage, a medicine, and an elixir of life.

Chapter 3 will be devoted entirely to the researchers of the past century who perceived a number of the mysteries connected with water, each following his or her own unique path. The knowledge they acquired through their quests was put into the service of the purification and regeneration of water.

3

Pioneers of Water Research

EVERY ERA HAS ITS own contingent of eminent scientists. Among them are those who stray far from the predominant trends and dedicate their lives to what seem to be unlikely pursuits; they are generally regarded as eccentrics. The originality of their ideas and their highly unconventional methods earn them the mockery of their contemporary intellectual luminaries (or those claiming that role). As for the well-established institutions, they simply ignore them. True pioneers are rarely understood, and therefore rarely acknowledged during their lifetimes.

This was the case for Viktor Schauberger, the father of modern water research.

VIKTOR SCHAUBERGER— BIOENERGY THROUGH IMPLOSION

Viktor Schauberger was born June 30, 1885, in Ulrichsberg, a village in upper Austria. His family, several generations of whom had devoted their lives to nurturing and cultivating forests, had as their motto: *Fidus in silvus silentibus*. This roughly translates into English as "Put your trust in the silent forests." Like his father, grandfather, and great-grandfather,

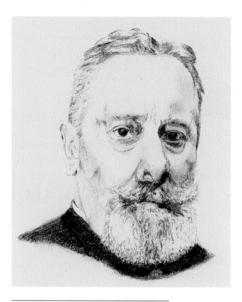

Portrait of Viktor Schauberger

Schauberger wanted to be a forester, but instead he followed in the footsteps of his brothers, studying natural sciences at the university.

A restless student, Schauberger rebelled against the tendency in universities to ignore the natural world and soon left to get a more practical education in forestry. He would later write the following lines, which were a radical criticism of both science and his culture.

The subdivision into categories of human intelligence is inculcated into children starting from the time they attend primary school. This has dramatic consequences, to wit, the extinction of creativity. It causes the human being to lose his sense of individuality and capacity for observation. Eventually, although he is a creature of nature, he becomes incapable of forging connections between the things he sees and the natural environment. The scientific objective is to create as nearly as possible a state of balance that is actually impossible to obtain, so it inevitably brings about a general decline of the economy. This is why the rules on which these activities are based are effectively erroneous, as they fit inside nonexistent parameters.

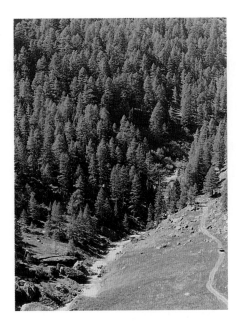

Water in its natural environment, a state of perfect balance.

What we should keep in mind is that the science of Schauberger's era was based on false assumptions. Scientists of that time were postulating the existence of stable situations. They believed they could resolve any problem (as Schauberger said, "balance it") once and for all simply by discovering the appropriate law of nature and applying it. To Schauberger this notion of nature presupposed a naive, utopian mind-set, one that is divorced from life's realities. He was utterly convinced this would have catastrophic consequences for society as a whole and its interaction with the natural world.

The Water Watcher

As a child, young Viktor had been able to watch the movement of water in a stream for hours at a time without ever getting bored. Over the years these living waters had surrendered all their secrets to him, one by one. This is how he eventually grasped all the understanding necessary to devise an ingenious system for floating tree trunks upstream. The engineers for the Water and Forest Department of Upper Austria could not comprehend how such a system was possible, so they hired an expert named Philip Forchheimer to accompany this extremely talented forester as he performed his duties. Schauberger was far from delighted at this prospect, but he consented, nevertheless, to reveal to this world-renowned expert in hydrology a little secret he had learned. In a book he wrote on the subject of water, Hans Kronberger recounts an amusing—and edifying—anecdote about these tutorial strolls in the forest. An abbreviated version follows.

One day Viktor Schauberger brought an eminent professor to the edge of a trout-filled stream and pointed to one fish holding itself motionless in the water, despite the very strong current. Obviously it was able to resist the pull of the current with little or no effort. Schauberger then extended his cane over the water in such a way that its shadow fell over the trout. It immediately swam away, against the current, to hide. The forester then asked the illustrious hydrologist if he could explain how the fish was able to do this: first remain motionless in the middle of a very strong current, then swim upstream against it. Met with the embarrassed silence of the engineer from the Department of Water and Forestry, Viktor Schauberger noted mischievously: "Well, Professor, it is because it was not educated in the university! If you had been in the swiftly flowing stream, you would have been swept away."

The technique that Schauberger developed for floating logs made it possible to transport large tree trunks against the current. The weight of these trees was far greater than that of the water, so logically they should have sunk. For the engineers of the Water and Forestry Department in charge of that area, such a feat was incomprehensible, but for Viktor Schauberger, there was a logical explanation for the phenomenon. All that was necessary was to apply the laws of nature as he had observed them.

Nature Is a Series of Dynamic Moments

Schauberger believed that nature is made up of dynamic situations—an uninterrupted series of dynamic moments. Everything in nature is in perpetual motion; one form evolves into the next, and new forms and conditions follow relentlessly upon each other's heels. Whatever we look at—an anthill, the sky, and so on—reality compels us to accept that it is subject to nonstop change. Nothing remains stable or balanced.

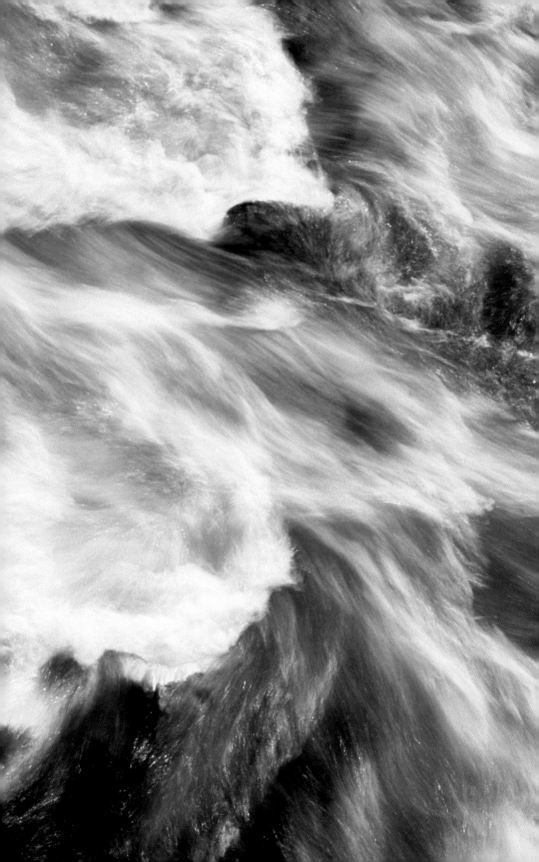

Hence the misguided nature of scientific criteria that insists on reproducing experiments that always have identical results. A more accurate perception of nature forces us to take into account the dynamic aspect of all natural circumstances and things and develop it into more comprehensive views.

Nature does not know airtight, securely compartmentalized categories like biology, chemistry, physics, and so forth. Schauberger was of the opinion that these categories could be found only in the human intellect and the hermetically sealed environment of a laboratory—never in nature. Human intellect is a handicap to the extent that it can only grasp things in a fragmentary fashion, as disconnected parts, which is not the way it exists in nature. He considered the mania for fragmentation to be the second major error committed by the official sciences of his time in their study of nature.

Movement and Energy Are Omnipresent

Since everything is transforming ceaselessly because it is in perpetual motion, it can be postulated that energy is present throughout the whole of the universe. In Schauberger's case, this deduction was a result of his tireless observation of natural facts, which allowed him to realize that everything exists inside a field of dual forces, each in constant opposition to the other: attraction/repulsion, condensation/expansion, concentration/dispersion. Without forces like these, the universe would be nothing but a shapeless, inert mass devoid of all life.

But what is the primary source of energy? What is the source of the instructions that keep it constantly moving and restructuring? Schauberger credited an omnipresent creative intelligence, a radiant energy capable of organizing all things by virtue of a primordial cause that was the source of all subsequent causes. He called this original energy "perpetually creative intelligence" (in German, ESI, for *ewig schöpferische Intelligenz*). It can be found everywhere in the universe, and its function is to maintain life within a creative, harmonious current, moment by moment. This is the fundamental principle upon which all of Viktor Schauberger's research is based.

Energy Production through Centripetal Compression

One of the major enigmas pondered by the young forester in his quest to unravel all the secrets of water was the ability of trout to leap over six-foot-high waterfalls and master a gradient of several hundred yards in order to reach the spawning grounds. His tenacity eventually bore fruit. One day he had a flash of realization that would become the starting point for later research when he suddenly realized that water—both in its falls (when unobstructed) and in its (natural) course—has a spiral, winding movement that allows it to generate a powerful energy at its center. It was at this exact central point that the trout would be found, the very place where the energy is simultaneously intensely concentrated and "at rest." This is how it was possible for these fish to remain motionless in the middle of very powerful currents as well as how they were able to get out whenever they wished, and even make leaps of six feet or more. This spiral vortex and centripetal concentration formed a natural source for collecting energy, a realization that eventually would make Schauberger's name synonymous with the principle of "energy production through implosion."

Using Pressure to Purify Water

When Viktor Schauberger examined the problem of cleaning waste- or polluted water and began devising procedures capable of restoring its fundamental purity and vitality, he based his efforts essentially on the principle of implosion. To everyone's astonishment, he succeeded in perfecting a treatment plant capable of restoring these waters to their original, crystal clear appearance. Not only did the process he created take little time, but it also required no electricity or the addition of any chemical substances. What was his secret?

In nature water does not flow in straight lines but follows a meandering, winding course. Hence the formation of spiral vortexes that both restore vigor and energy to water and disperse pollutants and other impurities that it may contain.

This is why Schauberger was so adamantly opposed to the adaptation and straightening of waterways. In his opinion, human interventions of this nature could have nothing but disastrous repercussions, as they deprived the water of its innate ability to regenerate.

Public works departments in Austria and a growing number of other countries are now paying more heed to Schauberger's discovery, which is a very good thing. But the errors that have been amassed over decades of ignorance are so extensive that correcting them now is extremely costly to taxpayers. In addition, devastating floods have resulted when waterways have been diverted from their natural course.

With the support of his son, Walter (1914–1994), Viktor Schauberger perfected various devices for the purification and refinement of water. The principle behind these devices consists of forcing the water through a complex circuit of pipes, funnels, and barrels, all of which have been arranged with extreme precision in order to impose ever more powerful and ever more dense, spiral, clockwise movements upon the water. The centripetal whirlpools formed in the water generate the phenomenon of implosion on the subtle plane. This imprints the swirling movement on the clusters of molecules that then fragments and simultaneously concentrates and "liberates" the natural bioenergy. This procedure restores the water's innate capacity to regenerate and rebuild its original structure.

As we shall see later in this book, nearly all the devices and systems currently available for revitalizing water work in accordance with a similar principle, even if the techniques or procedures themselves change from one appliance to the next.

A Tragic End

Viktor Schauberger was the target of much criticism and disparagement during his lifetime. Exacerbating this was the trauma of World War II and the confused situation in which Austria found itself immediately after the war. He accepted offers from several American industrial firms and moved to the United States. (I should mention that when the Russian troops invaded Austria, they sacked and burned his home.) His American adventure ended in disaster, which he found both painful and incomprehensible, and he felt as if he'd lost everything. Schauberger was a vision-

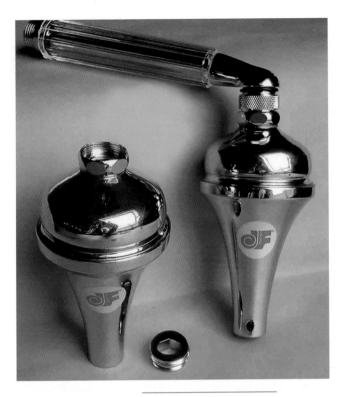

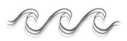

The authentic Martin water activator (based on the discoveries of Viktor Schauberger) is affixed directly to the water tap.

ary whose brilliant ideas had all been stolen, either directly or indirectly, often because he didn't want them used for military purposes. He was forced to sell his patents and died within days of finally being allowed to return home to Austria from the United States (September 25, 1958). For more information on Viktor Schauberger's water discoveries, visit www .schauberger.co.uk.

The Water Activator
according to Schauberger

After taking a seminar with Viktor Schauberger's son, Walter, engineer Wilhelm Martin decided to find a way to put the principle of water's spiral coiling movement, as defined by the senior Schauberger, into application commercially. The first water activator was sold as "the authentic Martin water activator." Initial diagrams were drawn up in 1972 at the Pythagoras-Kepler School in Bad Ischl, Austria, and the first model was produced in 1980. A German firm, Jens Fischer, took on the task of manufacturing and marketing the device. The authentic Martin water activator is now used in thousands of homes and businesses. By swirling the water it breaks apart the molecular clusters that are typical of dirty or polluted water. Water thus purified becomes sweet to the taste once more, and can again provide vital energy to human beings as well as to animals and plants. The most notable benefit this provides is the stability it guarantees the physical organism and, a fortiori (the stronger reason), the immune system.

SHOI YAMASHITA—VITAL WATER

After the death of Viktor Schauberger, research into the properties of water went into a long period of stagnation, at least in Europe. Japan continued the investigation, and there are two individuals who need to be cited here, namely Shoi Yamashita and Shinji Makino.

In 1964 Shoi Yamashita made the discovery that water from plants could be distinguished from ordinary water by its physical and biological

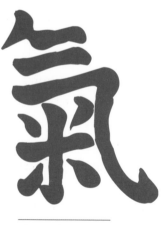

Chi, vital energy

properties, which could be compared to the cellular fluid of the human body. Yamashita dubbed this "living water" PI. PI is a term designating *qi* or *chi,* a Chinese word meaning "vital energy," but this PI is also akin to the perpetually creative intelligence identified by Viktor Schauberger. We shall revisit this concept in the next chapter.

Shoi Yamashita's plan was to find a way to transmute ordinary tap water into PI water. Like the discoveries of Schauberger (about whom he knew nothing, not even his name), those of Yamashita have their origin in his observation of the natural environment. The device he developed, with the assistance of Shinji Makino, was visibly inspired by natural processes.

The production of PI water requires putting tap water through the following three stages of treatment:

1. *Filtration.* Tap water is first sent through two different filters. The first filter, made of cloth, eliminates suspended particles in the water, as well as impurities such as rust and lime. The second filter, which is made from coconut bark, eliminates organic pollutants, herbicides, pesticides, chlorine substances, gas, and bacteria.

2. *Activation.* The lower part of the device that produces PI water is equipped with two ceramic spheres filled with calcium powder (made from fish bone) that are set into motion upon contact with water. It is these spheres that initiate the swirling movement that restores the water's vital energy (PI).

   The activation stage breaks apart unwanted molecular clusters that are created by the pollutants the water is carrying. The PI energy generates the impulses necessary for healthy and harmonious molecular groupings to form, groupings that conform to their original structure. The operation that breaks up the undesirable molecular clusters also has the effect of extending the inner surface of the water, which tangibly improves its ability to dissolve and form sound, harmonious molecular clusters.

3. *Energization.* The third stage of Shoi Yamashita's procedure consists of passing the water through a kind of miniature coral reef. It is known that coral encouraged the formation of life in the

primordial waters, generates mineral ions, and increases the pH of the water to an optimal degree. (It may not be coincidental that a good number of the inhabitants of the islands in the southern part of the Japanese archipelago live to the age of 120.)

After its passage through the coral reef, the water to be dynamized travels over a bed of carefully selected crystals taken from the peaks of Japanese mountains. These crystals invigorate the water and prompt its molecules to form harmonious clusters. The electrical conductivity of the water also diminishes significantly because of this, which stabilizes the new molecular structure.

Thanks to these three stages—filtration, activation, and energization—Yamashita and Makino's device is very effective for producing PI water—a prototype, to a certain extent, for the dynamization of water. Their work has been the source of much inspiration for amateur experimentation as well as stimulated extensive research by expert technicians and engineers.

ENZA MARIA CICCOLO— SACRED SPRINGS AND WATERS OF LIGHT

Biologist Enza Maria Ciccolo's interest in miraculous waters is partially coincidental. During a 1984 family vacation in the Pyrenees, near Lourdes, it occurred to her to take samples of the rock, water, and soil from the grotto. Her intention was to verify, through scientific analysis, if the water from Lourdes truly had therapeutic properties or if the healings attributed to it would not be more appropriately filed under the heading of superstition. She was also intrigued by the fact that germs and bacteria contained in the pools apparently did not spread.

On her return to Italy she entrusted her samples to a number of different laboratories, including one at the University of Milan. The analysis revealed that the water from Lourdes possessed a perfectly balanced electromagnetic field. We should recall here that particles of matter are in constant movement and that these movements take place around an axis. They move in one direction, either to the left or to the right, and this direction depends upon the charge, more or less, of the fundamental particles (photons, hadrons, and so forth).

In cases of a balanced charge, the number of rotations to the left and to the right are perceptibly equal. Rotations to the left pump energy out of the cells, whereas rotations to the right provide the cells with energy. In the event of an overload or disturbance in the electromagnetic field, the rotations toward the left will be predominant. This is the sign of an energetic imbalance, with repercussions on the molecular and cellular levels. In a relatively brief amount of time, this imbalance will deteriorate into a pathological situation. For example, analysis of the blood of a cancer sufferer will show a clear preponderance of particles rotating in a leftward direction.

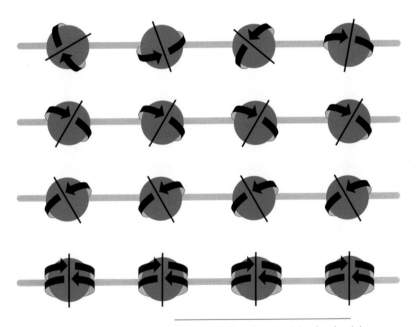

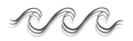

Top row: Chaotic rotations (and spin).
Second row: The majority of rotations are toward the right.
Third row: A preponderance of leftward rotations.
Fourth row: rotations (and spin) in balance.

Lourdes water, like other waters that have a reputation for performing miracles, "informs" and stimulates the elementary particles of a body that is ill in such a way that imbalanced rotations tend to regain their equilibrium. The initial laboratory analyses of the water from Lourdes, as well as subsequent research, gave Ciccolo a logical, scientific explanation for the remissions and spontaneous cures of "incurable" diseases.

Water Emits Luminous Waves

The question remained: What is the element that triggers the activity of the therapeutic water of Lourdes (or Fatima, or any other place with a high energetic potential)? What factor initiates the rebalancing impulse within a diseased organism? Ciccolo discovered that when the electromagnetic waves emitted by Lourdes water came into contact with pathogenic vibrations, they had the power to alter these vibrations, which reduced or eliminated the symptoms of the illnesses that corresponded to these vibrations. When contact with a miracle-producing water dissolved all the pathogenic vibrations of diseased cells or a diseased organ, it was a case of instantaneous healing. In other cases, the dissolution was only partial and the illness only diminished in intensity, thus beginning the healing process.

During the time of onset an illness betrays its presence by an imbalance on the vibrational plane and disruptions on the energetic, or subtle, plane. In contrast, an abscess, eczema, metabolic disorders, and so forth all reveal the ultimate stage of a disease.

The term *water of light* is justified in the sense that the water of a pilgrimage site is in harmony with the light, whether with all the colors of the spectrum or only a few individual ones. At Lourdes the water is in harmony with all the colors of the spectrum—undifferentiated—which constitutes white light. Therefore, the quality of the water of Lourdes is similar to that of white light. A number of scientists identify this quality of light with the essential energy of life. "Let there be light," as the Bible says in one of the first verses of the book of Genesis. In Italian these waters of light are known as *aqua a luce bianca* (waters of the white light). In the Germanic countries the term *marial waters,* referring to the Virgin Mary, is used instead. The first research on the properties of miraculous water used samples from places where there had been apparitions of the Virgin Mary.

Up to the present time, five hundred healings have been attributed to the water of Lourdes. The Catholic Church has not recognized all of these cures as miracles (it has only acknowledged about sixty-five). The last miraculous healing was in 1993 and involved a Frenchman named Jean-Pierre Bely who was suffering from multiple sclerosis. When he arrived in Lourdes he was almost completely paralyzed. Once he had been in the grotto, he recovered all his former mobility. This healing was confirmed by scientists and doctors who were members of the verifying body known as Comité Médical International de Lourdes. Bely traveled to Lourdes in a wheelchair but was able to board the train for his return unassisted, relying only on his own two legs, which had recovered their former strength.

Ciccolo undertook analysis of hundreds of different waters that were believed to possess special qualities, many of which had been taken from places other than pilgrimage sites. She determined that water of light could be found at these other sites as well, and that therefore the phenomenon was independent of religious beliefs.

This analysis of a multitude of miracle-producing water samples also revealed that there were different qualities of water of light. Some were in harmony with no more than two or three colors of the spectrum. These variations explained why some of the waters were suitable for curing gout or rheumatism, while others were appropriate for treating eczema or allergies. In other words, a certain number of waters that are described as waters of light have therapeutic properties that fit within certain proscribed limits. Ciccolo also observed that the active power of a water of light is not stable but can vary with climactic conditions. Additionally, some waters had a greater effect at night and on the days of a full moon.

The Prodigious Multiplication
of Waters of Light

As the result of her discoveries, Ciccolo developed a procedure for a kind of cloning of these waters of light. The procedure transmits the characteristics of a water of light into ordinary water. Nine drops of a water of light are enough to transfer its characteristics to a glass of tap water or a spring. The result is a water of light that is more or less similar to the initial water of light.

Ciccolo settled in Numana, in central Italy, where she opened a research institute and a healing center that offers treatments using water of light. There she is said to have performed miracle cures. She describes herself as a scientist, but she is also a visionary ahead of her time, just as Viktor Schauberger was ahead of his.

FRIEDRICH HACHENEY—
LEVITATED WATER

Friedrich Hacheney, born in Detmold in 1959, is the youngest among the researchers in the field of water regeneration. After graduating high school, he studied geophysics first at the University of Innsbruck, then at Munster University. His father, Wilfried Hacheney, an engineer who constructed water channel systems, had examined the innate properties of water during the 1950s. Like Viktor Schauberger, he understood the advantages of integrating coiling devices into water mains and other water transport systems and favored wood or other natural materials. He had long been aware that submitting water to pressure greater than a kilopond* incontrovertibly reduces the quality of that water. Only the activation of water through spiral coiling movements—a procedure used by ancient Romans in the construction of aqueducts—allows it to preserve its colloidal nature and retain its vitality.

---

*A kilopond measures magnitude of force exerted by gravity on a kilogram of mass. It has never been a part of the International System of Units (SI), which measures units of force in newtons.

Water's Ability to
Suspend Substances

Water's colloidal nature is its ability to transport substances in an optimal solution for proper ingestion and assimilation by the human body. A colloidal state is one in which substances are suspended. This colloidal property, which is an innate aspect of all healthy water, results from a force acting in opposition to the force of gravity. It is the force of levitation, or ascension.

Toward the middle of the 1980s, Friedrich Hacheney developed a device specifically for restoring this ascension ability to dirty or polluted water. The procedure consisted of causing the water to form precisely calculated whirlpools. The force that fractured the molecular clusters formed by pollution in this water created mini-whirlpools and mini-shallows so effectively that the water was able to restructure itself to be healthy and harmonious. This also enabled it to absorb oxygen more readily, becoming more vital and reactive.

Properties Confirmed by
Scientific Research

Over the past twenty years a number of studies conducted in collaboration with universities and other research institutes have corroborated numerous benefits of levitating water, including improved transport of nutritive substances in plants, increased detoxification of the human body, tangible reduction in limestone residues, improved bonding of cement and paint colors, and notably better results in germination of vegetables. The water levitation device developed by Hacheney is available commercially almost everywhere in the world. It is used to purify and enrich domestic water as well as that used for industrial purposes.

Levitated water intended for drinking is bottled manually in glass bottles. A number of large German cities have refilling stations offering levitated water for personal use.

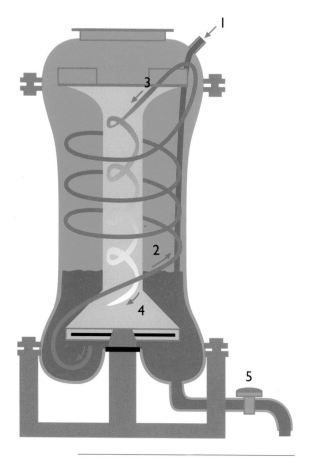

Apparatus for levitating water (developed by Friedrich Hacheney). Water enters the levitation machine at the upper right (1). Next, its movement is accelerated considerably by a suction rotor. The water then begins moving upward in a helix, spinning in a counterclockwise direction (2) before spilling into a central container (3). Here the direction in which it is spinning is reversed, and it begins moving downward. When the water reaches the bottom of the interior receptacle, it is flowing in an almost horizontal direction (4). At this point the water's movement is again accelerated by the reverse movement of the rotor. The speed of the water is now close to the speed of sound. The apparatus is then turned off and the water collected from it (5) no longer displays irregular molecular clusters and is devoid of organic impurities. It has recovered its innate ability to ascend.

JOHANN GRANDER—WATER ACTIVATED AND INFORMED BY MAGNETS

Man can distinguish healthy water from sick
water by its murmur and its burble.

JOHANN GRANDER

Johann Grander's techniques for revitalizing water have been successfully marketed throughout the world. In addition to its domestic use, Grander Technology (trademarked by the inventor) has found outlets in various industrial sectors. German steel mills, for example, use it to maintain the purity of the water used for cooling steel while simultaneously eliminating impurities. In swimming pools it allows for a significant reduction in the amount of chlorine additives required. And the Velden Casino in Austria uses Grander water to get optimal performance from its air-conditioning system.

The support of Austrian politicians and television advertising have both contributed to the success of the Grander label. Internationally, the Chinese use this water in the field of public transportation (some diesel locomotives are "nourished" with this water). In Europe, Johann Grander is considered to be one of the preeminent inventors of the twentieth century.

Genesis of the Grander Technique

The idea for this technique came to Johann Grander at a time when he had just resolved to change his life. This was in 1974, when he was forty-four years old. He had decided not to renew his lease on the service station he had run for many years, because he wanted to go back to nature. He began building log cabins, primarily in the alpine regions, to earn a living and support his family. He also built one near his home, as a kind of laboratory for his research and for tinkering on projects. Fifteen years later, he would realize a childhood dream—the purchase of a small abandoned factory called the "copper shack," which had long been used for extracting copper and silver. It was the precise location of natural springs that would later be used to produce the water that bears his name.

For a long time his interest was focused on magnetic phenomena, a passion he inherited from his father. He constructed, among other things, a generator equipped with magnets of a special alloy. When the generator was switched on, it produced a reciprocal stimulation of the magnets, creating a powerful magnetic field capable of generating very high frequency energy. He believed this machine could double the power of an engine.

His interest in engines quickly gave way to a passion for water when he observed that this high frequency energy, transmitted via a submerged battery, resulted in the relatively constant production of a water with very high vibrations. As often happens in scientific research, this fortuitous discovery ultimately resulted in his principal masterpiece.

The Grander Technique

The procedure developed by Johann Grander can be described as a bio-technical method of water purification and activation. Like the Martin water activator and the PI water-producing device, the apparatus developed by Johann Grander does not use electricity or require the addition of chemicals. The Grander device is encased in special steel and can be easily affixed to incoming water pipes.

Using specifically organized magnets, this apparatus causes water to vibrate at extremely high frequencies (around 100,000 hertz) and thus dissolve the molecular compaction that is characteristic of polluted water. The Grander procedure also rids water of its memory of pollution. Next, as in the technique conceived by Viktor Schauberger, the water is activated and energized by passing it through piping equipped with devices that cause it to form whirlpools along its route. Following this, the water passes into the proximity of chambers that contain a water with the ability to imprint its information on it. There is no direct contact between the two different waters, and no replacement of one for the other. Just the proximity of the Grander water is sufficient to harmonize the polluted water through its beneficial and therapeutic vibrations. It should be noted that the previous stages—magnetization and activation through swirling—have made it more

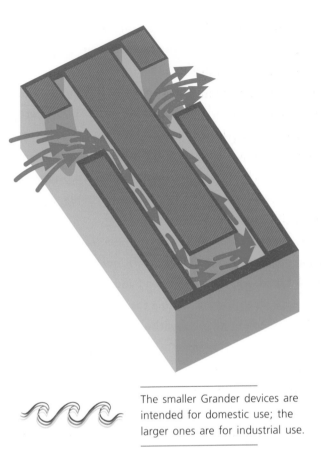

The smaller Grander devices are intended for domestic use; the larger ones are for industrial use.

sensitive in some way, making it more apt to take in healthy structuring information.

The vibrational effect of the informing water on the water to be "informed"—the dirtied or polluted water—can be compared in some way to that of a tuning fork. In a room where a certain number of tuning forks have been arranged, causing one to vibrate will cause all the others to vibrate. In this case the informing water transmits vibrations to the polluted water.

Enza Maria Ciccolo relied on the principle of resonance in her procedure for duplicating the waters of light. She poured several drops of a light water into a glass of tap water, using it as an informing water, so that the tap water began to vibrate at a similar frequency to the light water—an effect that lasts for a reasonably long time. To learn more about the phenomenon of resonance, refer to the boxed text in chapter 5 entitled "The Principle of Bioresonance" (page 115).

Grander water is sold in bottles via the Internet (www.granderwater .com), or you can buy tools for vitalizing water. For watering plants, the instructions recommend adding several drops of this water to a container of ordinary tap water. This will result in vigorous plants and magnificent flowers. Franz Alt, a German journalist and television newscaster, successfully applied this advice with very conclusive results, as follows:

> I placed two pots, each containing one grass reed, on my desk. The following spring, one had grown quite large, while the other remained small and scrawny. When I added several drops of Grander water to the water used in feeding the second plant, the results were astonishing: After only six months, the scrawny reed had caught up to the other in size and robustness.

In Austria the Grander technique is far from universally accepted, and although there are many who vouch for its properties, numerous others dispute it. On one side are those who rely on dominant scientific criteria and claim these properties are completely imaginary (including the dissolution of the residues of solid substances!). On the other side are those who confidently support the Grander technique (and those who have experienced spontaneous healing) but have not conducted a statistical inquiry. We have no trustworthy statistical data concerning the actual active principles of the Grander technique. It would be helpful to find out what the effects are and over what period of time from the more than two hundred thousand customers worldwide, for a more precise idea as to the extent and duration of the properties of this water.

Johann Grander is still alive but is living in retirement in his beloved Tyrol Mountains. For more information about the Grander technique, the reader will find it useful to consult the website referenced above.

4

The Power of Compressed Energy

We carried pitchers of water to the Tigris.
If we did not know we were fools when we did this
It is because we really are fools.

RUMI

THE PROCEDURES DEVELOPED BY Viktor Schauberger (water revitalized through implosion), Johann Grander (magnetic purification), and Shoi Yamashita (production of PI water) for the dynamization of water have inspired professional engineers, as well as a great many do-it-yourself handymen around the world. Their goal is to develop water vitalization devices that are even more effective than those mentioned above, or less costly. Various other apparatuses for treating dirty or polluted water have been developed in this way, and some perform as well as, or better than, those previously described.

There is no standardized vocabulary, alas, for this still new field of water vitalization and dynamization. It is therefore quite difficult to convey an exact idea of the way the different devices on the market function. Nonetheless, they all have one characteristic in common: they purify and activate water's essential properties without the use of any electrical current or the addition of any chemical products.

The energy that is responsible for the astounding performance and effectiveness of the different water dynamization devices is described by some people as natural, or vital, energy that transfers chi, or primordial, original energy. There are still others who use the terms *orgone* energy (first named by psychoanalyst Wilhelm Reich), or energy that has been treated with *tachyons* (hypothetical, speeding subatomic particles), both of which will be discussed later in the book. All these considerations are founded on incredibly complicated theories or notions that are extremely difficult to grasp, and not just for the novice. Personally, I use the term *vital energy* or *bioenergy* (a word derived from the Greek *bios,* which means "life").

I am now going to attempt a more thorough clarification of the concepts of regeneration and dynamization of water, as this is the objective of all the different procedures for treating dirty or polluted water that are currently available on the market. I trust that these explanations will also make it easier to grasp the principle at work in certain "miracles."

THE THERAPEUTIC PROPERTIES OF VITAL ENERGY

All natural therapies are intended to rid the human body of blockages that prevent energy from circulating freely and synchronize this circulation for the most beneficial effect.

In Chinese acupuncture, for example, the acupuncturist uses sterile needles to stimulate this or that path of energetic circulation (meridian) in the patient, an action that often relieves, or even eliminates, whatever physical or mental symptoms compelled the patient to seek medical assistance. But there are a large number of other therapeutic practices that seek the same result: special rituals, massage therapies, crystal healings, and so forth. Recently a device became available that seeks to achieve this same purpose by injecting the body of the patient with vital energy in a concentrated form. This new technique is akin to that of the universally familiar laying-on of hands.

The transmission of concentrated vital energy via the hands has been around since the dawn of time, used by many healers and shamans. A person who went to a healer for treatment would feel the energy spread throughout his or her body from the hands of the healer involved, accompanied by a flow of beneficial heat. This transmitted energy—or bioenergy—is capable of dissolving the energetic blockages in the person receiving it, rekindling dormant and wasted energies, and restoring energetic harmony in the individual's body and mind. Some healers also treat animals and plants. The effects are similar to those effected by the waters of light. Both are similar in nature to the phenomenon of implosion (Viktor Schauberger's technique for purifying polluted water) and any other dynamization procedure based on bioenergetic principles.

WHAT EXACTLY *IS* VITAL ENERGY?

Vital energy is omnipresent in the cosmos and consequently supports all organic life. The equivalent designations now most prevalent in the Western world are chi or qi, popularized by Chinese medicine and Eastern martial arts, and *prana,* which many people have learned of from Indian yoga. Hawaiian shamans call it *huna,* ancient Greece knew this vital energy as *pneuma,* and ancient Germans knew it as *Od* (a term designating the force that underlies and supports all natural phenomena). In the Hebrew tradition, we find the term *rouah,* which means "vital breath."

Sensitivity to vital energy is an aptitude that can be acquired quite easily. Anyone who would like to acquire this ability can begin by performing the following exercise: Sit outside beneath a tree with your back pressed up against its trunk. Allow yourself to totally relax, then fix your gaze on the silhouette of a tree in front of you, simultaneously focusing your mind and allowing it to empty of any stray thoughts. You should be seeing the tree in relief; in other words, really perceiving it as a three-dimensional object rather than a mental image, which is flat by definition. In a very short time you will witness the formation of an aura, or circle of light, around the tree, as well as spiraling whirls of luminous energy. What you will be seeing are bioenergetic manifestations. The radiant waves you may see flickering above asphalt roads on scorching hot days are also manifestations of this energy. Many people attribute this phenomenon to the overheated air, but they are mistaken.

To understand the relevance of this energy to the subject at hand, it is important to remember that bioenergy in a concentrated form is responsible for some bewildering phenomena. For example, many Westerners are somewhat skeptical when witnessing feats that Shaolin monks are able to perform, such as when a monk's head is struck with an iron bar, leaving the iron bar bent in half but the monk's skull with no signs of injury; or when they see a monk throw a stone with all his might at the chest of another monk without causing any harm to his rib cage. Exploits of this nature defy human reason. They don't fall into the category of sleight of hand, nor can they be ascribed to the muscular strength of the monks. The explanation is to be found in the stupendous power possessed by Shaolin monks to make themselves denser, to concentrate their bioenergy by means of a very strongly developed power of mental concentration. This requires rigorous training, which often takes many years. Powers as amazing as these are obviously not something that can be developed in one day's time.

The martial arts are based on a dual principle: strong internal concentration of bioenergy by the martial artist followed by the projection of this energy toward someone or something on the outside. There is no equivalent to the Eastern martial arts in Western culture, but we could stretch the parallels between feats of martial artists and those of a hero like Achilles in Greek mythology, or Siegfried in *The Ring of the Nibelung*. Achilles was eventually slain because an arrow pierced the heel of his foot, the single vulnerable spot of his physical being, the sole aperture in his energetic body. Siegfried's vulnerable zone was his shoulder, and Hagen, following Brunhilde's betrayal, pierced Siegfried with his spear in this very spot, thereby bringing about his death.

The fact that the West has long neglected or been unaware of the notion of vital energy has led to a very mechanistic notion of the universe. However, this very narrow-minded scientific perspective was thankfully partially abolished at the beginning of the twentieth century with the discoveries of Max Planck and his formulation of quantum theory.

In the domain of psychoanalysis the most fertile discoveries in the field of energy are attributable to Wilhelm Reich. The theoretical research he conducted on universal, vital energy, as well as the concrete applications he realized from this research, have become the cornerstone for a number of current techniques for activating and vitalizing water.

WILHELM REICH AND HIS DISCOVERIES ABOUT VITAL ENERGY

Wilhelm Reich was more or less a contemporary of Viktor Schauberger. The latter performed most of his work and research in the "old world," in Austria, while the bulk of Reich's activity took place in the United States.

Born in Austrian Galicia in 1897, Wilhelm Reich completed medical school in Vienna and became a practicing psychoanalyst there before moving to Berlin. In 1934, having been expelled from the Communist Party, he exiled himself first to Scandinavia, then in 1939 to the United States. In New York he practiced clinical psychoanalysis until he was expelled from the analytical movement. After this he continued his research, but as a completely independent scientist.

Wilhelm Reich was the target of extremely virulent polemics, undoubtedly more than any other scientist of his era. While some of his colleagues followed his work with interest, others furiously denigrated his activity. The former saw him as a genius, while the latter viewed him as a whiner with vaguely scientific pretensions, if not an outright charlatan. The ferocious opposition did not prevent Reich from formulating orgonomy, the science of orgone energy, which has been a springboard for a number of current trends in psychotherapy and natural therapies that are indebted to him. And, as I mentioned earlier, certain techniques used for the dynamization of water are also based on Reich's work.

For Reich, the term *orgone* is a scientific synonym for the universal energy of life. It is the energy that lends life to all living things and gives them their structure, both on the subtle plane and on the concrete, physical plane.

From Freudian Psychoanalysis to Vital Energy

As I made clear at the beginning of chapter 3, the research efforts on vital energy conducted by Viktor Schauberger are founded on his observation of water. But the passion Wilhelm Reich displayed for the study of bioenergy had a very different origin. In fact, when studying medicine at the University of Vienna in 1920, he frequented the circle that gathered around Sigmund Freud. He did not hesitate, however, to openly criticize Freudian psychoanalysis, reproaching it mainly for confining itself to the treatment of obsessive neuroses and hysteria that were plaguing a number of bourgeois Viennese women (which was the axis for the research of most of his colleagues). Reich considered this to be an elitist waste of definitive knowledge of the causes of mental distress. His interest was overwhelmingly drawn to the prevention of this suffering in children and adolescents as well as to the sexual education of adolescents. It was not long before he determined that both physical and mental health essentially depend upon unrestricted flow of vital energy through the musculature.

This was how he developed orgone therapy, the foundation for many current forms of psychotherapy that are based on the body and physical expression.

According to the explanations provided by Reich himself in *Die Ausdruckssprache des Lebendigen* (The expressive language of the living):

> Orgone therapy is distinguished from all other modes of influencing the organism by the fact that the patient is asked to express himself *biologically,* while spoken language is, to a great extent, eliminated. This leads the patient to a depth from which he constantly tries to flee. Thus one learns, in the course of orgone therapy, to understand and influence the language of living.

Reich used the phrase "to express oneself biologically." What he meant by this was "to display and live one's feelings without censorship"—to freely shout, weep, rant, explode in rage and anger, embrace, make love—

if the vital energy needed to be expressed in that manner, freeing it to restructure itself on a new foundation using different criteria. During Reich's lifetime, such energetic displays were considered extremely provocative. Reich, however, was deeply convinced that if vital energy were unable to express itself freely it would be incapable of assuming its true life-giving mission.

In essence, Wilhelm Reich and Viktor Schauberger were pursuing a similar objective. Both perceived that the process of purification and revitalization required dissolution of fixed, stagnant structures, which presumed going through a state of intentional chaos, a creation of negative vortexes and pathogenic energies, without which there can be no regeneration of vital energies or healthy restructuring.

A Noteworthy Biological Phenomenon

As a result of constantly listening to patients' words in his practice of psychotherapy, Wilhelm Reich became equally interested in the biological phenomena characteristic of the natural world. This exploration brought him into contact with some incomprehensible phenomena. For example, walking on the beach at night, he noticed tiny entities in the sand emitting a bluish light. When he put his hands in the sand, the rubber gloves he was wearing became charged with static electricity. As one might well imagine, this aroused his curiosity. He then had the idea of removing the light emission from any external influence, so he placed the minuscule entities into a metal box covered with an insulating material—a kind of Faraday cage. Now, to his great surprise, instead of vanishing, the luminous emissions intensified. What is more, spiral flashes had now joined the bluish "trails" that had first caught his attention. There was another thing that was even more astonishing: the protozoa continued to emit these flashes even after he took them out of the metal box. Looking at them under a magnifying glass, Reich obviously saw them enlarged, but he continued to see the flashes when he closed his eyes. What could be the explanation for such a phenomenon? It was only after detecting these same luminous "vapors" (which he would later name bions) in a blue sky in the middle of the day that he realized this energy also manifested in the atmosphere; that is, in the surrounding world. The phenomenon was of both a subjective and an objective nature.

The Science of Biophotons
for Measuring Vitality

A "photon" is a fundamental particle, a quantum of electromagnetic radiation, and the basic unit of light. Photons confer light (from the Greek *phos* or *photos,* meaning "light") and energy to all living things. Scientific instruments that make it possible to reproduce images of photons and quantify them are used, for example, to measure the vitality of a plant, a food product, or water. The term for the branch of science that specializes in their study is *biophotonics.*

Biophotonics originated with German biophysicist Fritz Albert Popp. In 1976, when Popp was conducting a series of tests at Marburg University with a doctoral fellow, Bernhard Ruth, he observed that biological systems give off light. He subsequently established that living organisms whose luminosity falls within the visible spectrum (between 200 and 800 nanometers) emit photons in a continuous sequence, which vary in intensity from several photons to a hundred photons a second, per square centimeter of the living organism's surface. It is the intensity of this photon emission that determines (approximately) the vitality of a biological system, such as a food product.

Tests performed on dynamized water indicate that almost all devices for revitalization that use concentrated bioenergy (orgone, chi, tachyons, and so on) intensify the emission of photons in the treated water. Consequently, it was not unusual to obtain water as pure as mountain spring water by using these devices. Regularly watering plants, grains, or vegetables with such high-quality water will increase their life expectancy and their shelf life. It is, therefore, no utopian fantasy to maintain, as some manufacturers of various water revitalization devices do, that drinking dynamized water is rejuvenating and increases well-being (even if these claims have not always been scientifically confirmed).

In writing about orgone energy, Reich speculated:

As children we used to be fascinated by the light phenomenon we observed with eyes closed: small bluish dots would move to and fro behind our closed lids. As we grew up, games like this lost their interest and we turned to other things. Adults lose confidence in their perceptions. Could we see the energy of the body this way—its biological energy—via our subjective visual sensations?

Accumulating Orgone Energy in Order to Transmit It

Little by little, Wilhelm Reich succeeded in giving more density to this orgone bioenergy by means of technical procedures. His central invention would be the orgone accumulator, a six-sided booth constructed of alternating layers of organic materials (to attract energy) and metals (to radiate energy), intended to capture and concentrate orgone energy.

Reich would use this captured energy for the treatment of illness, or simply to revitalize a patient. He maintained that humans, like other living organisms, are capable of capturing and harnessing this vital concentrated energy from the atmosphere, and of being regenerated by it. The majority of Wilhelm Reich's contemporaries viewed this as sheer idiocy and a flagrant denial of the progress that had been made by medical science over the preceding decades, and in the United States, the FDA ruled the accumulators a sham and ordered their destruction. Things have greatly changed since that time.

Recovering Health and Vitality with Orgone Energy

A number of contemporary health professionals use vital energy diffusers that are similar to the orgone accumulator developed by Reich.

Orgone energy restores the dynamism of a tired or ill individual's body, giving the immune system a much-needed boost. This energy can be felt spreading throughout the body; some perceive it as gentle, while others describe a burning sensation. In either case, the result is identical:

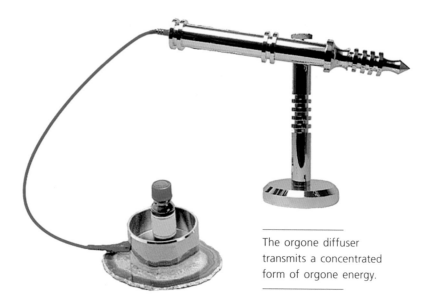

The orgone diffuser transmits a concentrated form of orgone energy.

a visible increase in the energetic potential of the person being treated. Some devices also measure the effect of the orgone energy in increased body temperature, both core and superficial (the skin), and accelerated heart rate. After a certain period of treatment—the length of which is determined by the needs of the individual patient—the lipids and/or cholesterol level are regulated, and there is even normalization of the sedimentation rate, a test that monitors inflammation in the body, which would indicate a strengthened immune system. Treatments with orgone also hasten the scarring of wounds and the healing of fractures, thereby giving the patient protection from certain complications. In the case of burns, orgone energy considerably reduces both pain and the formation of blisters and scars. There are countless case histories testifying to the therapeutic effects of orgone energy.

When reading this account of orgone therapy, it perhaps occurred to the reader that with several adaptations it could be used for the cleansing and purification of polluted water, or wastewater.

The process of the dynamization of water can therefore be defined as follows: it is the condensing and transmission of vital energy, otherwise known as bioenergy.

Ahead of His Time

When Wilhelm Reich published his discoveries on bioenergy, he turned the scientific institutions of the United States against him, if not the whole of American society. His work aroused sharp protest almost everywhere, and a relentless effort was launched to invalidate the man and his work, to a point where many regarded him as "mentally ill." He died in prison, where he was serving a sentence on racketeering charges (in an environment of general indifference), in 1957. (Viktor Schauberger died one year later.)

There is no evidence that the two seekers knew one another or ever even met. The fact remains, nevertheless, that both of them discovered (or rediscovered) the primordial, original vital energy. They both found ways to physically detect it, and both developed techniques for its use. In Reich's vocabulary, this energy, the "orgone," is the primordial creative energy that is omnipresent in the cosmos and responsible for the organization of all things and beings.

5

Bioenergetic Technologies for the Revitalization of Water

Ether, a subtle energy, is active in the forces of nature. Ether is the energetic tissue that underlies material forms and allows them to keep living. The interaction between ether and matter engenders all kinds of phenomena: inertia, mass, gravity, cohesion, and all the forces of nature.

PROFESSOR ADOLF ZIELINSKI

TREATING CROPS WITH CONCENTRATED orgone energy is a viable way of managing arable lands. The same procedure is being used to clean polluted waters, even some that are heavily polluted. Roland Plocher, a mechanic who is a native of Baden-Württemberg in Germany, is among the pioneers of this process.

THE BIOCATALYSTS
OF THE PLOCHER SYSTEM

While researching ways to reduce the devastating effects of certain pollutants, principally in agriculture, Roland Plocher had the bright idea of consulting the work of Wilhelm Reich. This was a fortunate decision as it led him to develop a procedure based on the principle of orgone enrichment and the holographic transmission of information. He tested the technique on heavily polluted surfaces, thinking it would help restore the soil's innate capacity of regeneration. He developed this process in the 1980s, in the large and lovely town of Meersburg, located on the shores of Lake Constance.

Plocher products didn't take long to start gaining international recognition. The principal sectors for their use are in the cleansing and revitalization of farmland, water purification plants, and larger bodies of water. The substance used in the method is quartz ground to a consistency as fine as flour, or a similar powder from another kind of rock crystal that has been treated with orgone energy. These finely ground rock crystals are like powdered fertilizers and act as a biocatalyst: plants become sturdier and more robust, and soil yield, as well as the quality of the grains or vegetables produced, improves. Plocher products also eliminate the need for pesticides, which, as we know, are essentially poisonous for both plants and for the environment. Lastly, Plocher products considerably improve water quality.

〜〜〜

The Goldau Zoo in Switzerland provides an excellent illustration of these claims. This zoo, like all zoos, is a heavy consumer of water. Water is required for quenching the thirst of the animals, cleaning their enclosures, and providing an environment in which they can frolic to their hearts' content. For this latter use, the construction plans of the Goldau Zoo included a pond that encompassed 12,400 square meters (14,830 square yards). All the buildings and surrounding areas in the zoo were designed to take advantage of natural light and the sun's rays. This has its

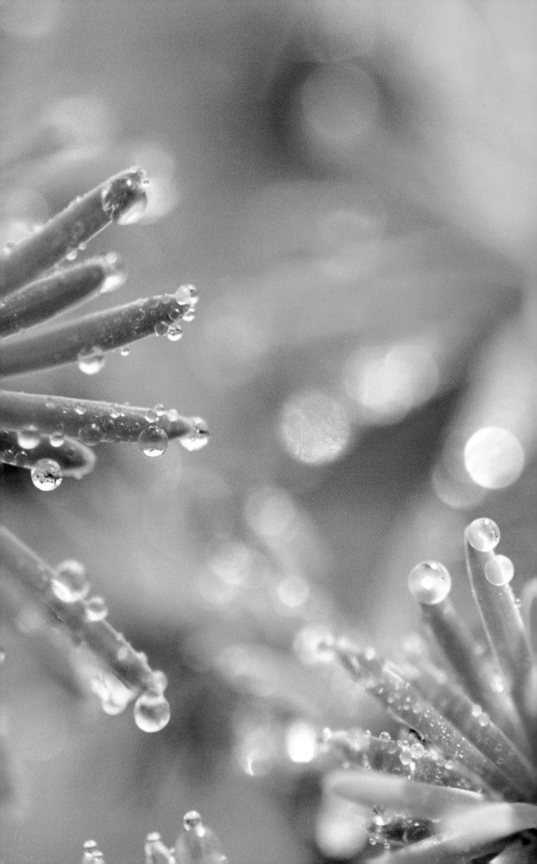

advantages, but there is also a down side: during periods of high heat, the water temperature would become too warm, resulting in a proliferation of algae. Cubes of feed and carrots—food that zoo visitors were permitted to give to the animals—would regularly sink to the bottom of the pond, where they decomposed. The wastewater was purified with sand filters; however, that did not preclude the need for regular cleaning. This involved a massive waste of potable water. The pool used by the bears had to be emptied once a month—sometimes every two weeks—because of the thick accumulation of sludge on the bottom.

In 1993 the Goldau Zoo signed a maintenance contract with the Roland Plocher company. The firm advised cleaning and regeneration using dolomite quicklime treated with orgone energy—which proved incredibly effective, as we shall see. The maintenance of the bear enclosure, for example, was now so simple a child could do it. In fact, it was enough to simply sprinkle one to two tablespoons of dolomite quicklime there each day. For cleaning the bottom of the pool, it was now necessary to empty it only once a year, and even then mainly to retrieve tools that had accidentally fallen in, or to remove rocks and branches.

Before 1993, all it took was two or three days of scorching midsummer heat for the wild boar pen to start emitting a foul odor. But once the zoo administration had signed the contract with the Plocher company, all it took was a sprinkling of 24 grams (approximately 0.8 ounce) of dolomite quicklime every week. This allowed the nitrogen to break down quickly and eliminated almost all risk of nauseating odors.

Finally, maintenance costs for cleaning water at the Goldau Zoo have plummeted. In addition, the animals seem to appreciate having their water purified by this dolomite quicklime. To quote journalist Joachim Andermatt in a recent article in the zoo newspaper:

> Previously, the ibexes would drink from mechanical watering troughs fed by spring water; now they drink water from the pool inside their enclosure. Animals have a sure instinct—they know what is good for them.

Scientifically Verified Results

There is scientific confirmation for the effectiveness of Plocher products. In fact, since 1993, the polytechnic college in Lower Saxony, Germany, has been performing a series of tests in three water purification stations. In two of these stations a distinct improvement in water oxygenation coincided with the use of Plocher products, which also reduced the cost of aerating the water by two-thirds. There was a similar reduction in the nitrogen content of this water.

Plocher products are even more effective in treating manure. Various testimonials indicate that they reduce its stench to a notable degree, or even eliminate it entirely. Only a small amount of product is necessary to achieve such results—the treatment of 100 cubic meters (130 cubic yards) of manure requires around a kilo (2.2 pounds) of orgone-treated quartz powder.

A second, equally convincing study, by a researcher named Adrian Nufer, was published in 2003 by a Zurich magazine. From a scientific perspective, the demonstration of the effectiveness of Plocher products is still in its infancy, but according to Nufer, their efficacy has been empirically proved. His study of their effectiveness in forest regeneration has a bearing on the multiple uses of these products. Nufer's website (www.nuferscience.ch) tells us this:

> Forestry is also faced with the problem of soil regeneration. Several decades of atmospheric pollution have greatly acidified the soil of our forests, which in turn has brought about imbalances of a hydraulic nature. Our forest floors now resemble desicated sponges that have become incapable of absorbing rainwater. Because the rise of underground water through capillary action can no longer be guaranteed, the forest floor is insufficiently irrigated at the surface. In addition, the mycorrhiza* are regularly damaged by nitrogen residue from the atmosphere. By creating long-term improvement in the quality of the

---

*A symbiotic connection between fungi and the roots of most plant systems; a critical link between root and soil.

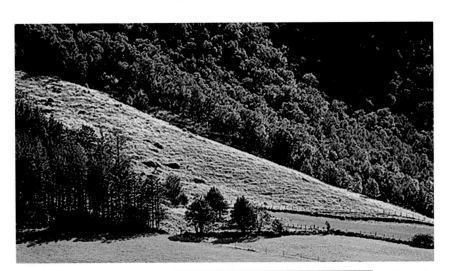

Reforestation helps restore hydraulic balance.

surface soil, and therefore also in the condition of the mycorrhiza, Plocher products provide a new and continually improving source of nutrients, which are furnished to the trees by indirect fertilization. This restores their strength and stamina, and thereby increases their powers of resistance. Furthermore, the application of a special compound has facilitated the reforestation of formerly unsuitable terrain. This is particularly valuable on the very steep slopes of high mountains, where such reforestation helps to protect against avalanches.

A Simple but Brilliant Principle

One might ask how such extraordinary remedies are constructed. The masterpiece of the Plocher system consists of a collecting funnel that is several yards tall.

The energy collects at the bottom of the funnel in a kind of narrow corridor formed by two plates of glass and containing a specific substance, which could be oxygen (the information contained by oxygen informs the carrier material, which is beneath the glass plates). This phase of the energetic intensification of the support material in which it receives the information can last from ten to twenty minutes. The carrier material should be selected in accordance with the ultimate intake—quartz powder,

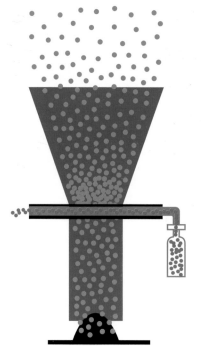

The Plocher device: Free bioenergy in the atmosphere accumulates inside the collector where it becomes "denser," like orgone. The orgone becomes saturated with information (a holographic form of transmission). The shapeless orgone "informs" the carrier material (such as quartz powder).

powdered magnesium carbonate, stone, or other. The material selected should have a rough, uneven surface.

The use of this support material that has been informed by oxygen and treated with orgone does two things: permits a notable dynamization and catalyst for all biological processes (this is the action of the orgone) and leads to the formation of a much more substantial quantity of oxygen.

Initially the traditional scientific establishment considered this process to be far out and crazy, if not downright dangerous. Roland Plocher actually received his inspiration from a procedure commonly employed in ancient Egypt (and also used by the Celts), one that later also inspired the master builders of cathedral bell towers.

This inspiration was the *djed* pillar, a column with four capitals that the ancient Egyptians invested with divine power. Priests customarily tied bundles of grain around these columns, convinced that this would guarantee better preservation of these grains. A number of current researchers view the djed as an absolutely fantastic orgone collector.

As I mentioned earlier in this chapter, the device developed by Roland

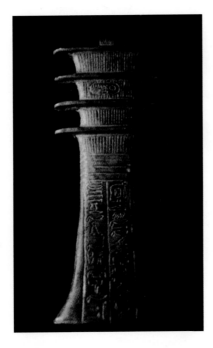

The djed of ancient Egypt

Plocher has earned an international reputation, and this was accomplished without any kind of public subsidy or grant.

REVITALIZATION OF WATER WITH GEOMETRIC SHAPES—THE WEBER BIOENERGY SYSTEM

While attempting to develop a procedure for collecting bioenergy and transmitting it into dirty or polluted water without any kind of carrier substance, which would then trigger natural biocatalytic processes in the water, German engineer Eckhard Weber discovered the beneficial action of specific geometric shapes. He constructed brass rods in accordance with the laws of sacred geometry, then covered them with several layers of protective sheathing. The rods come in several different sizes and are installed on water pipes (see illustration on page 86), but they can also be immersed directly into the water. He patented the process using a product called the Weber-Isis Water Activator.

The Weber-Isis Water Activator restores the harmony of the atomic and subatomic fields of polluted or wastewater and uses a biocatalyst to free its vital energy. A Shauberger water activator can be placed alongside it

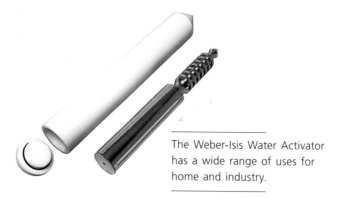

The Weber-Isis Water Activator has a wide range of uses for home and industry.

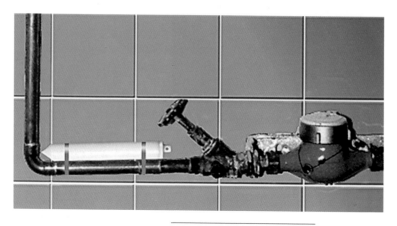

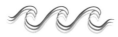

The Weber-Isis Water Activator can be mounted on a water pipe with a hand tool. It should be placed in close proximity to the elbow, with its point directed toward the vertical pipe.

("upstream," so to speak). It is recommended that both of these activators be placed on the water intake pipe.

The Weber-Isis Water Activator has earned its own international reputation. It is used for a wide variety of different purposes and locations: cleaning of lakes, water purification stations, hotel industry, restaurants, car washes, dairies, gardening, fish hatcheries, swimming pools, bottling of water and fruit juice, and so on. It comes in different sizes to accommodate the varying amounts of water requiring treatment.

The Weber-Isis Water Activator softens water and tangibly increases its reactivity, but it also hastens the breakdown of the aerobic bacteria that are gluttons for oxygen. It greatly reduces the proliferation of pathogenic germs and bacteria and absorbs even the worst odors to such an extent that even the most polluted wastewater can be restored to its best quality. The Weber-Isis Water Activator also prevents the proliferation of cynobacteria (better known as blue-green algae) that occurs so frequently in lakes and ponds. Lastly, it helps break down organic muck (sapropel, from the Greek words *sapros* and *pelos,* which mean "putrefaction" and "mud," respectively) and excess nutritive substances. In these cases, the device is attached to a rope and then immersed in the water to be treated—a lake, water purification station, and so on. As Eckhard Weber noted:

> The use of Isis Water Activators for the cleansing of lakes and ponds is a tricky business. In fact, acid rains, manure, the various substances used for crop protection, and periods of scorching heat all contribute to the rapid deterioration of our aquatic environments. Furthermore, the number of Water Activators required must be carefully calculated, based on the number of cubic meters of water to be treated.

In developing countries where it is used to purify water or keep wells and reservoirs potable, the Weber-Isis Water Activator is valued highly.

The effectiveness of this device has been confirmed by numerous blood tests performed in (independent) laboratories. The two photos that follow clearly demonstrate its effect.

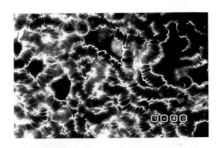

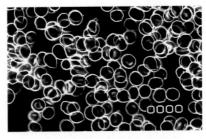

You can see how strongly the platelets bond together here: the subject drank tap water.

Here the image of the platelets is almost normal. The test subject drank tap water that had been revitalized by a bioenergetic process.

Now, in order to help the reader get a better grasp of the distinctive characteristics of the Weber technique, we need a short digression into the domain of sacred geometry.

Geometric Shapes with Therapeutic Properties

Ancient Egyptian civilizations had a profound knowledge of the therapeutic properties of the shapes inspired by sacred geometry, as can be seen in the construction of their pyramids. For example, if you were to reproduce a miniature version of the pyramid of Cheops, scrupulously respecting the proportions, and place food inside it at a precise spot, you would see that this food would last longer than food stored randomly. Shops specializing in the esoteric sciences sell pyramids for precisely this purpose, as well as for their therapeutic properties, or for creating more intense states of consciousness. Anyone visiting an Egyptian pyramid who is even a little sensitive to the waves emitted by shapes will quickly feel an expansion of awareness. Because of their proportions, some shapes have the innate property of capturing orgone energy and therefore possess the ability to restore harmony to the surrounding environment.

The fabled scientific knowledge of ancient Egypt was carried over the Mediterranean to Greece, home of Pythagoras, who is more frequently credited for mathematics. Many people are, in fact, unaware that he was initiated by an Egyptian priest. On his return to Greece he opened a mystery school. All manner of sciences were taught in this school, including the cosmic laws of cosmogony and geometry, which enable the harmonious organization of the universe. What interested Pythagoras were less the geometric figures in and of themselves than the establishing of cosmic order (the famous golden mean,* for example) on earth through the example they offered. His theory served throughout the Middle Ages as the basis for construction of both sacred and commercial architecture. He inspired not only the master builders of his time but also the builders of Romanesque and Gothic cathedrals. Various city squares and other spaces

---

*The golden mean, or golden ratio, expresses the idealized relationship of two parts of a whole to each other and to the whole. It has been used extensively in both art and architecture.

were also laid out in accordance with the laws of sacred geometry, creating spaces with an intense, palpable energy.

Among American Indians and Asian peoples the most widespread sacred form is the mandala. The primary function of a mandala is not decorative, as many Westerners imagine. Every mandala is a depiction of unique, cosmic, celestial organization. It represents both material and nonmaterial realities and is intended to give the order and energy of heaven a concrete presence on earth, by means of meditation and rituals. This holds equally true for yantras, the geometrical equivalent of the mandala. The energy of a mandala or a yantra is just as powerful as that of a perfectly proportioned Egyptian pyramid, or certain Romanesque, Gothic, and Baroque buildings.

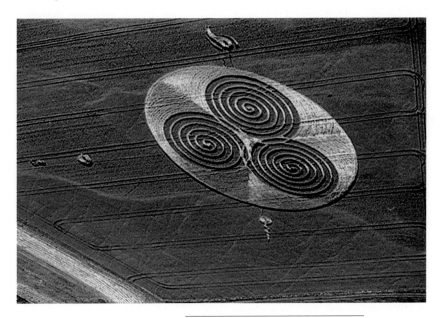

Crop circle mandala, Calden, Germany (2000)

Synchronization of Energy Fields

Sacred geometric forms emit powerful beneficial vibrations, the potency of which depends on their size and orientation. Vibrations of this nature pass into the surrounding space (and everything within that space), where they have a therapeutic effect. In addition to its balancing effect on water, the Weber-Isis Water Activator transmits synchronizing, beneficial vibrations into the environment in which it is placed. It is thus able to neutralize the effects of electromagnetic radiation, disruption caused by water veins, cell phone signals, and so forth.

Neutralizing Car Exhaust

In this context, it is worth mentioning at least one example of the many experiments performed with a Weber-Isis Universal Activator, especially since this account is particularly revealing of the device's potent effect. To perform this experiment, two diesel cars were parked in greenhouses of equal size. Every day for a period of several weeks, an employee turned on the engines and let them run for half an hour. Both cars were exactly the same except for one difference: a Weber-Isis Universal Activator had been fitted to the fuel pipe of one.

As a result of this experiment, all the plants died in the greenhouse where the car without the Weber-Isis Universal Activator was parked, whereas in the greenhouse holding the car equipped with this activator, all the plants were still alive. They were, however, covered with a fine film of oil, easily removed with a squirt from the hose. The noxious emissions had been neutralized by the vibrations emitted by the Weber-Isis Activator. Perhaps someday in the near future the Weber-Isis Activator or a similar appliance will replace the current catalytic converter. If so, it would also reduce fuel consumption from 5 to 10 percent. Diesel motors thus equipped would no longer bellow dark clouds of smoke. Although a Weber-Isis Activator can be pricey, it could eventually pay for itself. Installation is quite simple, and the unit comes with complete instructions.

To quote Horst Kohler, president of the Federal Republic of Germany: "Germany must become a land that is fertile with ideas." It seems to me that the Weber-Isis Activator is a brilliant idea, especially since it reduces

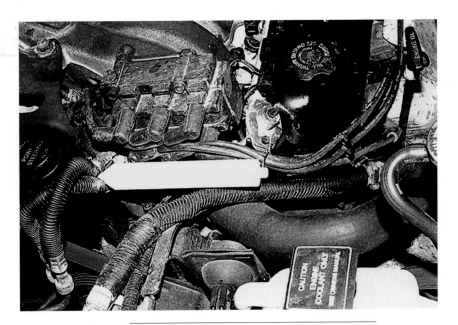

Fitting of an Weber-Isis Activator on the diesel motor of a car

the harmful effects of pollution. So it is deplorable that an inventor like Eckhard Weber is being harassed by competing companies that allege he is practicing unfair competition. Weber was recently forced to destroy large piles of his advertising brochures on the pretext that he did not sufficiently draw consumer attention to the official stance of the natural sciences, which maintains that orgone energy, or subtle vibrations, have no basis in reality. Consequently, there is no acknowledgment of the impact of orgone energy or vibratory fields of subtle substances on people's well-being.

It should be stressed that in Germany all companies that make orgone energy available commercially are mandated by law to include statements of this nature with their products and advertising. Some manufacturers evade this requirement with linguistic ruses, or by simply omitting the word orgone in their prospectuses or on their Internet sites. In its place they use neutral terms such as "natural energy" or "new technology."

Eckhard Weber has successfully held his own against vehement allegations from this pseudo-scientific Inquisition (there is no other word for it). Today he employs more than four hundred people in a number of different countries, and an increasing number of engineering schools have offered to scientifically test Weber's discoveries both on the theoretical plane and in concrete applications.

ALVITO: A SOLUTION
FOR ALL YOUR WATER PROBLEMS

In many respects the genesis of the Alvito Company in Nuremberg, Germany, resembles that of other manufacturers and marketers of water dynamization devices. Its inventor developed it based on lessons he learned from a difficult experience—a life lesson—but while his inspiration was not drawn from some well of universal knowledge, he is quite educated in this domain.

Inspired by Plocher

Hans-Helmut Preisel, a mechanical engineer, created the Alvito Company. Over the course of his life he had to deal with severe health problems, and his doctor warned that if he did not make radical changes to his lifestyle, he would have to undergo risky surgical interventions. These words did not fall upon deaf ears. Preisel decided to leave his business and began to take an interest in alternative therapies and holistic health. In 1992 his interests expanded to include biophysical methods for revitalizing water when he saw a German public television broadcast (ZDF) entitled *Wenn der Wassermann Kommt* (When the water man comes). From this he learned how Roland Plocher was regarded as the savior of lakes and ponds on the verge of turning in to open sewers, including even some that had already reached this stage of pollution.

Beyond making a great impression on Preisel, this documentary also sparked his creative genius. It gave him the idea of developing a device for "restoring order" into cellular life, starting with his own body. The success of his early efforts encouraged him to communicate his discovery to his circle of friends and acquaintances. At this time—it was 1997—with his son Harald he formed the company Alvito: Gesundheit und Umwelt

Gmbh.[Health and environmental factors incorporated] in Nuremberg. It has a vast product distribution network throughout Germany, and its reputation has gone far beyond this country's borders.

How the Alvito Water Vitalizer Works

Like every other dynamization device, the one offered by the Alvito Company does not use electricity or require any chemical products whatsoever. As explained in more detail in the box entitled "Types of Water Filters" (see page 97), it can be used in combination with an active charcoal filter. It can be fitted onto water pipes (for example, beneath the kitchen sink), and its installation is extremely simple.

Like the Grander process for dynamizing water, the Alvito water vitalizer uses the permanent magnet technique. Permanent magnets, you may recall, have the ability to break up molecular clusters and destroy the water's memory, thus rendering it sensitive to more harmonious configuration, which is healthier and life-enhancing. A meticulously defined arrangement of different magnets is what makes the Alvito water vitalizer so effective.

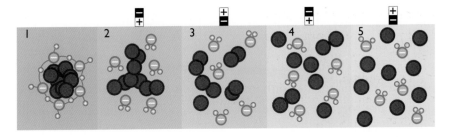

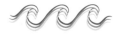

1. The water molecules encase the particles of impurities or polluting substances.

2. The magnets imprint a spiral swirling movement on the water molecules by means of their alternating charges. These whirlpools, or vortexes, break up the molecular clusters. This also removes the water's memory so that it is able to "forget" the structure imprinted upon it by the impurities and pollutants.

3. and 4. The molecules of the pollutants are also subjected to spiral vortexes, which cause them to break down into their constituent elements.

5. Because the water molecules are now liberated and vital, they combine differently, in a harmonious way.

The prospectus that comes with the Alvito brand water activator tells us this: "As a result of swirling micro-movements engendered by the magnets, the devices and the products are reprogrammed by a physical procedure; in other words, through the impulses imparted to them by other structures in the form of 'ultra-fine vibrations.' These vibrations, thanks to the principle of resonance, are communicated into the water."

Because I still had questions, I asked to meet the inventor's son, Harald Preisel, who was gracious enough to furnish me with all available clarifications about the basic principle. This is what he told me: His father had developed an apparatus capable of generating powerful and harmonic bioenergetic fields, to which he added an organic substance— green clay—that he left to be reacted upon over a certain period. This had the effect of creating a balance on the atomic and subatomic levels, thus engendering a symbiosis with the bioenergetic field mentioned above. In the Alvito system it is this treated green clay that is integrated into the water vitalizer. By virtue of the principle of resonance, the green clay communicates the characteristics of its electromagnetic field into the tap water, along with its mineral vibrations. Preisel added: "The atomic universe is a little like a vast concert hall where thousands of people are talking and singing, each in his own little world. But the orchestra conductor has only to step up to the podium and all these people come together as one under the direction of his baton. The result of this is a sum total of fabulous energy and a marvelous synchronicity, or harmony."

The Alvito Company offers an extensive range of products: personal care, household, water vitalizers, rings for water activation (washing machines, dishwashers), biodegradable laundry powders, and so forth. These products have earned a loyal base of customers, some of whom have been literally enchanted by their experiences with Alvito products. I would like to cite the testimony from one customer, Jutta Thomsen:

> For the last year and a half, I have been managing a hotel on the
> shores of the North Sea, a region in Germany where the water is

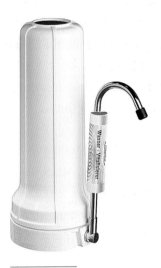

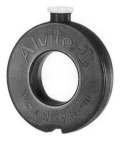

Alvito dynamization
ring for a washing
machine or dishwasher

The water vitalizer is
attached to the water
intake pipe or to the
main water pipe. (It
can also be combined
with a special apparatus
equipped with an active
charcoal filter, like the
device pictured above.)

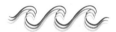

especially hard. It causes a great deal of problems for our electrical appliances; for example, the lime slake has a nasty tendency to clog up the electric boilers. Need I say more? Another annoying thing is how the laundry powder has trouble dissolving in this water, and therefore leaves streaks on white linens and bright colors. Our tiled floors can only be cleaned, and our tap water can only be made drinkable, by using huge quantities of chemicals and lots of elbow grease! Luckily, thanks to Alvito products, annoyances like this are now behind us, which has made the maintenance personnel much happier. The hours needed for cleaning have been sharply reduced, the quantity of cleaning products needed has been greatly reduced, and the dishwasher has stopped gobbling up salt and detergent. The plates and dishware are gleaming and the glasses shine. A pleasant odor of cleanliness now lingers everywhere, in place of the formerly dominant harsh and detestable chemical smells.

We have been using Alvito products for our laundry as well. For a machine with a fifteen-pound capacity, one cup of powder is more than enough; not only does it get everything extremely clean, it also smells good! Colors retain their brilliance and the linens are now soft to the touch. All the used water is free of chemicals and there is no longer any need to transport extremely heavy containers of water. Our customers rave about my "North Sea Champagne." I have also noticed the difference in the quality of the water in food preparation. Vegetables miraculously become green again in this water! This is extremely helpful, especially for green salad.

Water treated with Alvito products acts like a fountain of youth on women, both inside and out. It makes skin smooth and supple. There is no more need for expensive body creams with all their exaggerated promises!

Lastly, Alvito technology has amazing effects on cut flowers. Flower bouquets last three times longer. Cut roses now last up to three weeks.

The dynamization of water based on the Alvito process clearly transforms ordinary tap water into a "water of light," to borrow the term used by Enza Maria Ciccolo But wouldn't this be a somewhat rash, even completely idealistic assertion? On one hand, there are all these high-tech devices that require years and years of research and design. But we are suddenly witnessing the appearance of extremely simple devices like the Alvito and the Weber-Isis Water Activator. I would wager that both the extremely technical and the extremely simple devices have a bright future. Didn't the electronics industry have an equally humble and small beginning?

Types of Water Filters

Opinions are divided as to the actual effectiveness of the different water filters currently commercially available. Among the most effective at eliminating most of the pollutants in a safe and efficient manner are reverse osmosis and active charcoal. These involve a procedure of passing the water through a group of extremely fine membranes, or pores, which mechanically hold back the substances in suspension, or in solution in the water. The undesirable substances intended to be held back this way are numerous and varied and include bacteria, heavy metals, pesticides, chlorine, pharmaceutical residues, and so on.

Reverse osmosis uses filters with almost microscopic pores that hold back nitrates and minerals held in solution in the water and let nothing through but the water itself.

In the process that involves filtering through a pad of active charcoal, the filter is a bit rough so that it can allow the transit of the salts and minerals that are essential for the human body; this means that somewhere between 4 to 8 percent of the pollutants get through. This procedure has the advantage of stabilizing the pH of the water in such a way that it does not turn more acidic, which is a frequent side effect of filtering water through a reverse osmosis system.

(For more information about filtering water, see the section in chapter 6 entitled "Should Tap Water be Filtered?" on page 129.)

WATER VITALIZED BY TACHYONS

As most readers of this book are aware, bioenergy is very different from electrical energy. It is not of the world of electrons but of the world of the quanta, of fundamental particles (photons, mesons, tachyons, and so on). As we know from quantum physics, this world is governed by different laws from those that preside over the world of matter.

Quantum physics starts from the principle that there is no such thing as purely objective consciousness. In fact, it postulates that the observer, through the act of observing, transforms what is observed in some way. The laws of classical physics, therefore, do not apply here, as the assertions of the observer are necessarily subjective and of a speculative nature. This aspect of quantum physics is applicable to a water revitalization technique that uses the fundamental particles known as "tachyons."

This particular technique is the primary expertise of an American named David Wagner, who is extremely well versed in electronics. He is, in fact, responsible for the commercialization of bottled water dynamized by tachyons and bottled water of light. Several drops of these waters are all it takes to revitalize and purify dirty or polluted water (from the water table, aquarium water, a backyard pool, and so on). David Wagner's company, Advanced Tachyon Technologies, also offers silicon plates treated with tachyons for the dynamization of beverages, as well as other products and comestibles.

David Wagner's "Tachyonization"

As we have seen, bioenergy can be produced and collected in a variety of ways: sacred geometry (sanctuaries, mandalas, and so on), water implosion (Viktor Schauberger), orgone collector (Wilhelm Reich), funnel-shaped orgone collector (Roland Plocher), and so on. Now we will look at a procedure for revitalizing dirty or polluted water through the action of tachyons.

Using precisely arranged magnets within a special chamber, David Wagner produces a stable bioenergetic field that is harmoniously structured on the subatomic level. The characteristics of this chamber are passed along over a period of time into the object or substance that has been placed inside it. All kinds of objects and substances can be treated in this way: clothing, cosmetics, and water, to mention but a few. The tachyon energy, which has no "spin" and is not affected by vortexes or gravity, rebalances the item's subatomic structure and stabilizes its spin. These effects are capable of lasting for years, and objects or substances that have received this treatment will communicate their beneficial vibrations to the surrounding environment. Wagner has given a name to this procedure, which he calls "tachyonization."

Wagner's reputation can be attributed to the extremely original nature of his invention. He maintains that his procedure for dynamizing water not only develops a harmonious subatomic field of very high frequency but also generates tachyons. Tachyons, in his view, act as a kind of antenna to energy, the boundless cosmic intelligence with which, we might say, we are in direct contact. Wagner's theory about tachyons corresponds to Viktor Schauberger's concept of "perpetually creative intelligence." Tachyons (from

Tachyons: Hypothetical Particles
or Tangible Reality?

Do "particles" that are faster than the speed of light actually exist? The theory of the quanta created by Max Planck, then adopted by Niels Bohr and Werner Heisenberg, is founded upon the assumption that subatomic particles are neither solid nor separate entities from each other. Rather, they are energetic structures in continuous interaction with each other. What we call "mass" would, in the final analysis, be nothing but extremely concentrated energy, or more correctly, a temporary structure of frozen waves. Physicist Oliver Crane published the results of his own research in this field in 1960, taking it a step further with his opinion that neither empty spaces nor intervals exist. In this regard, we should make it clear that the ratio of scale between the surface and the core of an atom is more or less equivalent to that between Madison Square Garden and the flame of a candle. Could what we call matter be nothing more than intervening space? The answer is no. According to Crane, currents and vibrations of a mechanical nature fill the immaterial spaces. This is the true nature of reality: a vast ocean of energy in which all things are connected, as mystics from every tradition have maintained since the beginning of time. Physicist Gerald Feinberg was the first to postulate the existence of tachyons, in 1964. In 1991 Christian Monstein demonstrated the existence of currents of magnetic quanta-space. In the eyes of certain scientists, this alone was sufficient proof for the existence of tachyons, but others chose to regard it as merely an indication of their existence, albeit a decisive one.

the Greek *takhys,* meaning "rapid") are the interface between limitless space (the vacuum, ether) and solid energy (mass), thus they also offer a means of linking forms. This interesting theory is a bold one, to say the least, but one that is beginning to be influential. In any case, it makes it possible to grasp the notion of vital energy—a mysterious phenomenon—from a new angle.

Dynamization of Water Using Tachyon-Treated Fiberglass

There are a number of European companies marketing tachyon products for cleaning water. One of these is Abeiez Tachyon, a German-Swiss firm that sells rolls of tachyon-treated fiberglass. The fiberglass is wrapped around the main cold water pipe and affixed there (necessary materials are supplied at the same time the fiberglass is purchased). To ensure effective dynamization of the water, at a minimum, a two-foot length of the pipe should be wrapped with this fiberglass. The installation is as easy as it is quick and takes no more than five minutes.

The fiberglass is easy to transport, so it can also be used for outside events like festivals and parties, in tents, and so on. It is also sold in longer rolls for multifamily homes.

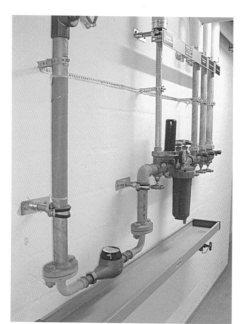

Tachyon-treated fiberglass wrapped around a water pipe activates and vitalizes the water as it travels through.

THE CHI ENERGIE CARD: A BIOENERGETIC COASTER

This "mini-disc" is not for your computer—it is a clever coaster for energizing water. You can use it at home, in the office, or in a restaurant and always drink the best water. The card has a silicon layer embossed with special bioenergetic information that picks up vital energy (chi) like a parabolic mirror. It concentrates and radiates it in a radius of about three feet. The concentrated chi energy harmonizes fields of destructive and aggressive vibrations of molecules, electrons, atoms, and quanta.

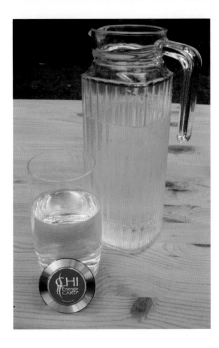

The Chi Energie Card

When you place the card under a glass, jar, or bottle, the water molecules immediately begin to rebuild their natural crystal structure; within seven minutes you will have soft, energized water that tastes very smooth. If you use it to make coffee or tea, any bitterness is reduced. Whether or not you prefer the taste, your personal energy level will rise when you drink this vitalized water. Placing the card under a bowl of fruit or in the vegetable drawer of your refrigerator will help these water-containing foods stay fresh longer.

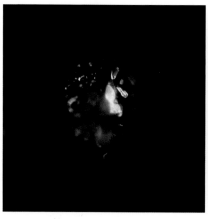 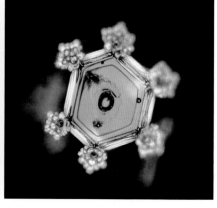

A drop of water, before vitalization

A drop of water vitalized by the Chi Energie Card (magnified 5000x)

Using vitalized water will heighten and balance your life energy. In Eastern philosophy chakras are energetic "wheels" in the body that absorb universal life energy and transport it to the organs and cells of the body. Take a look at the charts on page 103 of chakra and aura analysis before and after drinking water energized by the Chi Energie Card.

REVITALIZING WATER WITH CRYSTALS

Readers who eschew high technology for more natural methods of activating and revitalizing water will be happy to learn (if they do not already know) that there is a technique suited to their preference. This technique uses specific crystals selected for this purpose because of their energetic qualities.

Crystals have been a source of fascination since time immemorial, and there are two good reasons for this. One is their beauty, and two is their useful, or beneficial, properties that are as varied as they are impressive. To mention but a few: the energy collected in quartz provides the exact time to millions of people all over the world; laser rays and rubies are known for their effectiveness in dissolving bile stones; and needles coated with quartz are used in acupuncture.

Crystals store vibrations, but they also hold micro-information. We

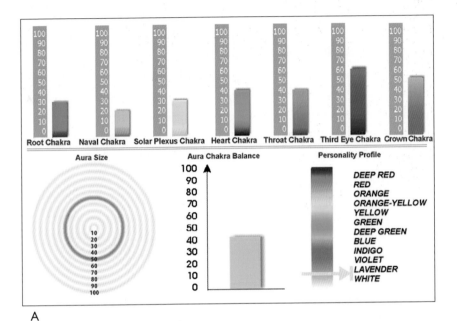

A

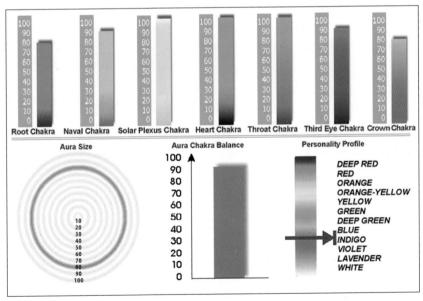

B

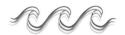

A computer-based chakra and aura analysis of a person before **(A)** and after **(B)** drinking water energized by the Chi Energie Card

should recall here that everything in the material world has its own specific vibration (wave length, frequency) and that we have instruments that allow us to measure them.

Each variety of crystal has its own vibratory characteristics and possesses a unique "sound." Silica, a major component of crystals, is what primarily collects vibrations. When a crystal comes into direct contact with water or is in close proximity to a natural spring, that water will absorb the crystal's vibrations and will in turn be absorbed by the individual drinking the water.

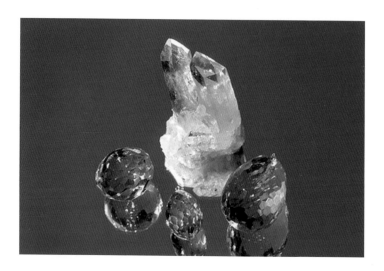

Preparation of Crystal Water

Anyone can easily create crystal water. The first step is to select a small crystal (or crystals) and place it in a container of water to which salt has been added (preferably sea salt or Himalayan salt), as a kind of purifier. Allow the crystal to soak in this water for about a dozen minutes, then expose the crystal to sunlight, which will increase its energetic potential. While waiting, pour fresh water into a pitcher or carafe, then carefully stir the water in a clockwise direction with a wooden spoon or rod. This will imprint a swirling movement, like a spiraling coil upon the water. It will now absorb the subtle vibrations of the crystal when it is placed in the water.

Crystal water can be drunk on its own or used for cooking or making tea. It can also be used to revitalize wilting plants. Crystal water should be consumed the same day it is prepared. It is recommended that this water not be exposed to direct sunlight.

Crystals used in preparing crystal water should be cut and not contain any rough surfaces. A smooth surface prevents germs and bacteria from being trapped and proliferating in the water. Many New Age shops and occult bookstores offer a wide selection of crystals. One or more may be selected either by trusting your intuition or based on your knowledge about crystals. Following is a short list of stones recommended for their healing properties or other benefits.

- Agate refines perceptions and stimulates the intellectual faculties.
- Rock crystal purifies the aura and supplies energy.
- Amber bestows wisdom, equilibrium, and patience.
- Jasper encourages dreams and stimulates the libido.
- Opal generates psychological stability.
- Quartz regulates the circulation of energy in the body.
- Rose quartz restores balance and dispels negative influences.
- Sardonyx is invigorating and therefore resists depression.
- Tiger's eye encourages the balance of the two cerebral hemispheres.
- Topaz purifies the aura and restores the joy of life.
- Tourmaline awakens love and increases sensitivity to spiritual forces (see page 106).

I personally have some experience of drinking water prepared using rose quartz. I drank water prepared this way for a period of two to three weeks. After this time I felt my aura had absorbed the energy of the rose quartz and that I was benefiting from its protective and rebalancing properties. The action of a crystal will vary, it is true, from one person to another. It is up to individuals to try this experiment personally and learn for themselves.

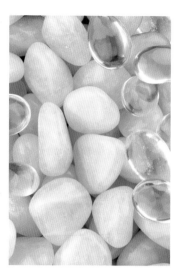

Tourmaline creates crystal water that increases sensitivity to spiritual forces.

Crystal water is widely used throughout Europe. In Austria, for example, there are a number of hotels that supply each guest room with this water. A pitcher of water is placed on the nightstand with several semiprecious stones or crystals alongside it. Most guests are delighted by this thoughtful gesture. In fact, when they return to their rooms exhausted after a long day of skiing or hiking, they are reinvigorated by drinking this crystal water. Many of the hotel guests are fully aware of the beneficial effects crystal water can have on body, mind, and spirit.

Crystal water is also used in agriculture. The Bonhausen family, for example, has a farm and orchards on the shores of Lake Constance. They collect rainwater and pour in spring water containing crystals and plant extracts. As agricultural engineer Margit Holland wrote:

This recipe is one that we (the family) perfected by trusting our intuition, which guided us to reconnect the water and the fruit trees.

The rainwater was put into a creek lined with quartz sand, which has a reputation for its ability to store sunlight. This energy was then transmitted to the water running over the quartz bed of the creek. The result was extremely positive for the trees, their foliage, and the quality of their fruit.

Holland added:

Other fruit-growers who took great care of their trees but were unaware of the importance of water had trees that were not as sturdy and vigorous.*

Some water activation and revitalization procedures integrate crystals in a very targeted fashion. The selection of the stones can be made intuitively or by relying on disciplines such as radionics or kinesiology to produce a water that matches the individual customer's desire most closely. To illustrate this, I would like to cite two procedures for purifying and energizing water with crystals, one marketed by the Pichler Company, the other developed by Gebhard Bader-Donner (the Elisa Energy System).

Water Purification
Using the Pichler Procedure

Revitalization of water with the Pichler device uses a mixture of ordinary and semiprecious stones that are selected in accordance with the customer's actual needs. The Pichler company sells two kinds of products

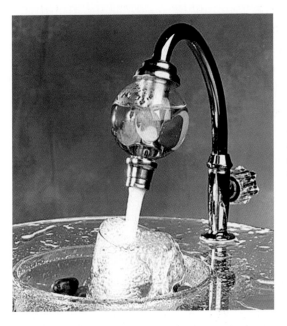

A Pichler water purification device

that complement one another but can also be used individually. The basic principle, however, is the same in both cases. The water intended for treatment is poured into a coiled tube in order to imprint a swirling movement upon it, thus purifying it, after which it is run over a bed of carefully selected stones. Inside the Pichler Water Ball is a golden coil that is used for revitalization, whereas the spiral of the main device is ceramic (and made by hand).

The Elisa Energy System

> *Building a water installation is much more an act of meditation than of physical science.*
> GEBADO (GEBHARD BADER-DONNER)

Gebado is the nickname for Gebhard Bader-Donner, the inventor of the Elisa Energy System. Without question, he is one of water revitalization's foremost champions. Furthermore, he places great emphasis on making only unique pieces. Each piece is the result of the infinite sum of his knowledge and his vast experience.

Elisa water revitalization devices are carefully tailored for each customer and designed to respond to that customer's specific needs. Before doing anything else, the person installing the system will arrange a meeting to discuss the desired characteristics of the system. The basic installation is then performed in accordance with one single principle: the water is first whirled through custom-made stainless steel sheathings. This several-stage procedure eliminates most of the pollutants in the water and causes it to lose its memory of these harmful substances. The water next travels through hermetically sealed crystal chambers containing gold nuggets, minerals, or other substances with high vibrational frequencies. A layer with a synchronizing resonance made of local pine wood, which is itself sheathed in high-quality copper, provides the finishing touches for the crystal water funnels. The majority of the parts used to carry the water are manufactured from stainless steel of impeccable quality. Some of these systems have the capacity to treat close to two hundred and fifty gallons of water an hour. If the customer so desires, the company can also install an integrated filter system that uses active charcoal or reverse osmosis. This serves as an additional precaution to catch any potential residues, particularly heavy metals.

The following testimonial was written by Andreas and Christina Fischer-Colbrie of Mondee, Austria, and provides one example of the many satisfied Elisa customers.

During the month of October in 2002 we purchased an Elisa water revitalizer, and this system soon became our pride and joy. Many bakers preceded us in taking this initiative, and, like them, we cannot help but talk about the splendid results. The dough rises better and never gets close to a risk of fermentation, and the

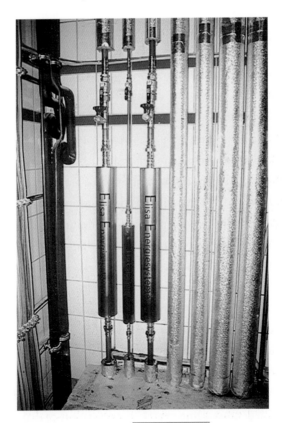

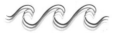
Elisa installation for swirling crystalline water in a bakery

machines have a much higher output. Even our first-year apprentices are enthusiastically citing the amazing quality of the dough we now produce in this way. We have also noticed that the ovens and water pipes do not collect scaling anywhere near as much as before.

But the essential improvement is to be found in another place entirely. It lies in our rediscovered family harmony; the installation of the Elisa water revitalization device marked the start of a brand-new life. Ever since that day positive events have followed one upon another without interruption—there have been more in the last few months than over the past thirty years combined. Such health and harmony among three generations living under the same roof is extremely positive. This energy is also transmitted into our business, where it has worked wonders and been the source of the creation of numerous new products.

Gebhard Bader-Donner has a complex, almost metaphysical perspective on water. He writes:

Something that seems incomprehensible at first turns out to be nothing more than an optimum imitation of natural processes. Even as a child I felt myself irresistibly drawn to stones and water. In the eyes of a child, water seems like a magical substance. For example, whirlpools fascinated me and I was never happier than when I let myself get sucked into one. Adults considered games of this nature to be quite risky. Quite frankly, I would advise against them as well, had I not emerged from them unscathed. Many years later, in my therapeutic work, water appeared to me as an essential key. A divine power. Without this key, we cannot go forward.

Doctor Gottwald Schmidt, whose practice is in Bad Reichenhall, Germany, studied crystalline water that was processed with an Elisa Energy System and made the following observations:

Water is an exceptional substance. The human body consists of 80 percent water, so we should pay close attention to the water we drink. With respect to the Elisa-process crystalline water, its most notable effects can be attributed to its strong reactivity.

Its capacity for bonding with oxygen is more substantial than that of other waters. Its absorption of pollutants and wastes is better, thus their elimination through the kidneys, liver, and skin is also better. Elisa crystalline water stimulates cellular activity and strengthens the body's innate ability to erase the information connected with pollution (an ability it shares with homeopathic remedies) . . .

Another characteristic trait of Elisa crystalline water that supports the health of an organism is its direction of rotation (clockwise), which has the effect of enhancing all therapeutic activities, of whatever nature (bioresonance, magnetic field therapy, homeopathy, music therapy, color therapy, and so forth).

REMOTE WATER DECONTAMINATION

Bioenergetic, or orgone, shapes crafted in accordance with the laws of sacred geometry as well as tachyons and crystals are powerful means for purifying water but are sometimes insufficient for decontaminating large bodies of extremely polluted water. There is, however, a recently developed technique for activating and revitalizing water that is even more effective than those previously mentioned. It consists of injecting the polluted water with complementary therapeutic information that has been very carefully perfected. The technique is known as radionics.

Put as simply as possible, radionics is a process of remote healing. The study of this specific method for the purpose of revitalizing water began several dozen years ago. While we don't have space here for a complete history of this sector of scientific research, I can provide a basic outline. Radionics is based on the following presupposition: all life-forms share the earth's electromagnetic field, and each life-form also has its own "blueprint," or "morphogenetic field," that determines the way it behaves (this is true for the human, plant, and animal kingdoms).

The best-known pioneer in the field of radionics is Rupert Sheldrake, an English biophysicist.

Morphogenetic Fields: Energetic Blueprints

Sheldrake's research began with an account of a singular behavior that appeared one day among a flock of tits (similar to the chickadee) in Southampton, England, in 1921. In those days it was customary for milkmen to deliver fresh bottles of milk to homes and leave them by the entrance. One day these birds began alighting on the milk bottles and opening them with their beaks so they could drink the milk. It was then noticed that the birds were clearly following the milk trucks on their delivery routes, and once the milk had been left, swooping down and enjoying a little feast. This extremely singular phenomenon kept spreading farther and farther afield. We are fairly well informed about its development after 1930. We know, for example, that it eventually spread to eleven different species of birds but was first and foremost passed among the different varieties of tits.

Tits never fly too far from their nests—fifteen miles at most— and even that would require exceptional circumstances. As this behavior extended much farther than fifteen miles, observers were forced to acknowledge that it did not involve the same flock seen in Southampton. Was this possibly a coincidence? The phenomenon continued to spread and at one point was noted in Holland, then Denmark and Sweden— all a considerable distance from the first place this behavior had been observed.

With the outbreak of the Second World War, milk deliveries to individual homes were interrupted and did not resume until 1947. By this time all the tits who had been alive before the war were now gone, but this didn't stop the phenomenon. Observers had to accept the fact that the birds' descendants had adopted the behavior of the previous generation. The whole process—identifying the bottles, taking off the lids, enjoying the milk—was imprinted in the memory of the tit family of birds. It was, so to speak, inscribed in their genes.

Sheldrake's studies of the similar spread of behaviors among other animal species led him to formulate a hypothesis of the existence of morphogenetic information fields for an entire variety, or species, of living things.

The presence of a blueprint of biological phenomena has been confirmed by means of Kirlian photographs (photographs of the energetic fields of living beings). By way of illustration, a Kirlian photograph of a fragment of a leaf restores that leaf to its integral wholeness. A single piece is all that is needed to restore the entire energetic field that underlies a material form. The energetic field of a material form survives its disappearance or annihilation, and we have techniques for reproducing it.

This would explain why someone who has suffered the amputation of an arm or a leg continues to have the physical sensation of this limb and even be able to feel pain in this phantom arm or leg that no longer has any physical reality. That limb continues to exist in the form of electromagnetic vibrations.

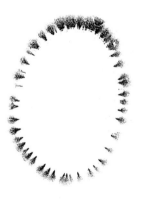

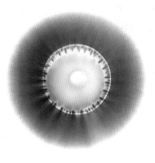

Kirlian photograph of ordinary tap water

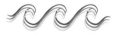

Kirlian photograph of the same water after it has been treated by a water revitalization process (in this instance, the Weber-Isis Water Activator)

Modification of the Energetic Blueprint

The studies conducted by Rupert Sheldrake imply that morphogenetic fields change with the development of knowledge. Some behavioral patterns vanish from an animal's energetic blueprint to be replaced by new ones. I would like to cite Sheldrake's tests with rats in this regard. These experiments permitted him to observe that each successive generation of rats placed in a water maze were able to discover the exit more quickly. Without moving any rats, researchers in other countries, including some quite far away, were surprised to note that the rats they were observing in a similar labyrinth had acquired the same knowledge. It was impossible for the transmission of this knowledge to have a genetic origin, for the simple reason that these rats had never had any contact with those observed by Sheldrake.

We have now reached an utterly fascinating stage in behavioral research, and we could, by analogy, pose the question in regard to the transmission of information to polluted water or wastewater. By what means do waters like this learn to behave differently, and how can they be inspired to reorganize themselves on a new basis? The answer is: by means of the principle of biophysical resonance. This principle has already been brought up, readers will recall, several times in this book.

Cleaning Large Bodies of Water by Means of Informational Data

Some instruments permit us to detect and measure the resonance frequencies of a substance. What they actually measure are the oscillations between negatively charged ions and a positively charged core. In this sense, we could say that morphogenetic fields are an electromagnetic phenomenon that can be detected and read by electrotechnical devices that are capable of dealing with them in a direct, targeted fashion. This brings us back to the principle of radionics, a procedure that is used to clean large bodies of polluted water.

One of the leading companies for radionics is M-TEC, with corporate headquarters in Altenkirchen, near Munich. Quite recently the company designed a system that connects to a computer and scans the morphogenetic fields of water for therapeutic purposes. All the water in an entire

The Principle of Bioresonance

Let's imagine a vast concert hall in which a number of string instruments have been placed. What would happen if the note "A" (440 hertz) were played on one of them? All the strings tuned to the A note would immediately start to vibrate, precisely by virtue of the principle of resonance.

In order for two things to resonate together, they must fundamentally be "on the same wave length." For water, this is the case when a water of light, or informational water, comes into contact with another water. The informational water establishes resonance with the other water that has dead or latent vibrations. The result is a change in molecular structure. (Johann Grander, for example, contends that ordinary tap water, when establishing contact with an informational water, remembers its original substance and recovers its intrinsic vitality.)

lake can be analyzed from a single drop, because, as I explained earlier, this drop contains the integral wholeness of the morphogenetic blueprint of all the water in this lake. The electromagnetic vibrations that have been scanned in this way allow the computer to detect any symptom complex and suggest a treatment in the form of compensatory vibrational frequencies. The principal data bank used here is homeopathy.

The frequency models for cleaning a large body of water are fine-tuned using various technical procedures to transmit graduated waves into the water drop that has just been analyzed. These waves represent therapeutic information that is valid for the morphogenetic field of the entire body of water. This may seem completely crazy to some people, like something out of science fiction, but the results indicate otherwise. Readers of this book should not be surprised, especially if they recall the preceding sections on water of light, or the informational water of the Grander label.

Cleaning a Lake in Berlin

In 2000 the municipal council of Berlin voted approval for cleaning Dreipfuhl Lake (Berlin-Zehlendorf) and entrusted this extremely delicate task to the company of Mundus GmbH. Dreipfuhl is a completely enclosed lake of around two-and-a-half acres in size.

The lake was in deplorable condition—its large sludge content stopped its water from regenerating properly because of the deficiency in oxygen and heavy metal pollution. Residents of the neighborhood regularly sent petitions to their elected representatives complaining about the extremely foul stench that flooded their neighborhood because of the lake, especially after hard rains. When the already heavily polluted water of the lake absorbed additional pollution from street runoff, dead fish and algae would cover its surface. Dreipfuhl Lake experienced an environmental collapse of this nature two or three times a year.

The municipality studied several proposals for cleaning the lake but found most too onerous or difficult to be implemented. The town officials finally decided to have the lake cleaned using a radionic technique. Given the results, I cannot help but congratulate them for their choice.

The first stage for cleaning Dreipfuhl Lake consisted of installing three energy generators (known by the name of Prige) in its waters. The Prige generator collects orgone and transmits it into the surrounding water. The introduction of a sufficient quantity of bioenergy to an expanse of polluted water restored the water's ability to self-regulate, as the effect of a biocatalytic process.

In the second stage of the cleaning of Dreipfuhl Lake, the water was infused with extremely targeted information of a therapeutic nature. In order to do this, the M-TEC company proposed a radionic approach (like the one just described). The company began by taking several samples of lake water, scanning their electromagnetic vibrations, then comparing the results with those obtained by laboratory analysis of the same water. The two diagnoses matched to an amazing degree. The therapeutic program drawn up by the computer (which matched one drawn up by a human being) was the following:

➤ A homeopathic preparation based on eucalyptus, white clover, Tabacum, and Urtica Crenulata. In human therapy eucalyptus is indicated for respiratory disorders; white clover for circulatory problems, thrombosis, embolism, and even constipation; Tabacum is effective against delirium, dizzy spells, and blackouts; Urtica Crenulata is used to treat itchiness, hives, allergies, and skin eruptions.

➤ In the sphere of organotherapy the rectum (waste dispersal) as well as *ventriculus cordis dexter* (right ventricle valve) were indicated.

➤ An assortment of minerals and semiprecious stones (carefully selected with an eye to their vibrational frequencies).

- Chrysoberyl (known for its purifying properties)
- Limestone or Icelandic crystal spar (a pure, crystallized version of calcite)
- Jasper (also known for its purifying properties)
- Meteorite, high iron content (rebalances pH, among other things)
- Rhyolite (generally prescribed for inflammation)
- Turquoise (known to strengthen gums and teeth in humans)

The choice of remedies clearly showed that the company was not interested solely in treating a morbid process but rather a living, holistic system. Water that has been dirtied or polluted cannot be revitalized in a satisfactory manner using mechanical remedies.

The company M-TEC treated the water of Dreipfuhl Lake on the morphogenetic plane. This measure, combined with basic energizing techniques, healed the lake in a relatively short time. In just six months it was clear once more and its water was transparent. It had recovered its auto-oxygenation capacity (including during times of high heat). People no longer saw dead fish floating on its surface. Aquatic plants were again growing normally, both at the bottom of the lake and on its shores. The flora was healthy once more. Samples taken by independent experts confirmed that the level of pollutants, mainly the heavy metals, had diminished considerably in the lake water. To cite one example, the chrome content before the cleaning took place was 2.38 mg/l and was now no more than 0.015 mg/l. Needless to say, no chemical product of any kind was used in this cleaning operation, and mud was no longer accumulating on the lake bed. For those unaware of the therapeutic effect of regeneration procedures for polluted water, results of this nature must appear little short of incredible!

In fact, the cleansing of Dreipfuhl Lake retriggered biological processes that, in some way, taught the water how to change its behavior. I should add, however, that the city of Berlin also took steps to reduce factors causing the pollution, thereby showing respect for the lake (which it was due), as well as compassion.*

The example of Dreipfuhl Lake in Berlin allows us to extrapolate that radionics can help clean even larger bodies of water—for example, inland seas. We may one day learn that even the waters of Lake Baïkol or the North Sea—which today more resemble open-air sewers than natural bodies of water—have been regenerated. The required funds for projects of this scope would hardly exceed the postage stamp budget of a government department. The obstacle is, therefore, not financial. We have the means to annul the effects of human unawareness of the natural environment.

HEALING MOTHER EARTH
AND HER WATERS

In the course of my research for this book, I came upon a very personal account of an unusual water healing that I'd like to share with you in closing this chapter. It illustrates the way in which spirituality and modern technology can work hand in hand. This is what Christan Hummel wrote:

Very few among us can deny that we are living in exciting times of change. The new millennium is filled with thoughts of hope as we prepare to embrace a new era, as well as some fears of that change.

---

*I learned of this from an article that appeared in *Hagia Chora,* the geomancy magazine I cited earlier—issue 14, 2002.

The environment is teetering on the edge. Violent storms and changes in weather patterns, sun flares and magnetic fluctuations continue to remind us how very alive and dynamic our Earth is, and how much our survival depends upon her.

Although I cannot see into the future, I do feel in my heart that the intensity, severity, and even complete possibility of the earth changes predicted can be changed. And the experiences I, and hundreds of others, have had in recent years support this view.

Nature's Hidden Intelligence

Some of the ways she has given to participate in this transformation of hers are in the area of environmental changes. This began for me back in January of 1997 in my work with a man named Slim Spurling. I discovered through dowsing that I could use that as a way of communicating with the hidden intelligence of nature, known to me as the devas, and that with this newfound tool I could take that relationship from the simply subjective into the more objective world of the dowser. With that tool the devas themselves jumped on the opportunity to show us how they wanted to work with us with the new tools we had discovered.

One of the new tools we were working with was an energy device developed by Slim Spurling, called a Harmonizer. He and his partner, Bill Reid, had been utilizing these tools that are based on zero point technology and have amazing effects on individuals and on the environment. We witnessed many miraculous events with these tools, but what interested me the most were the applications to the environment. Through sound and sacred geometry the Harmonizer was able to clear pollution in Denver, Cairo, and Mexico City in test cases.

New Technology Depends on User's Intuition

What was interesting about the Harmonizer was that it was a different kind of technology that depended upon the intuitive abilities of the user. Of course our meditation background helped here. We would tune in to Mother Earth and ask from our hearts for the best

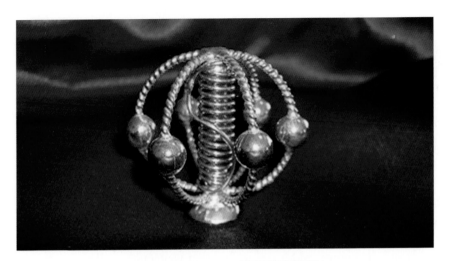

Harmonizer

time and location for the Harmonizer to achieve maximum results. It seemed that this added significantly to what they referred to as the "tuning" process. We discovered that by first asking Mother Earth about the location and time of use, the results surpassed what we observed when we relied only on the hardware of the technology. When we added the element of working with the devas and dowsing for what and how they wanted the Harmonizer used, it shifted things to a whole quantum level.

Clearing Geopathic Stress

After working with the Harmonizers in this way in various other cities and seeing similar results, I was convinced that this third-dimensional reality was able to be influenced in ways I'd never conceived of before. In one instance in the Salton Sea the air pollution was so bad that we couldn't see the mountains only ten miles across the water. We used the Harmonizer and asked the deva of the Salton Sea how to work with this tool. We were shown to offer the blueprint, or thoughtform, of the Harmonizer and the frequencies of the tape being played to the deva and told that it would be able to reproduce it. Within ten minutes we saw the pollution clearing in front of the mountain before our eyes!

While there, we also worked with the devas to do a clearing of the geopathic stress of the area. Before we started I dowsed for the geopathic stress lines in the area, and they were every couple of inches apart. During the clearing process, which took about thirty minutes, we offered the deva some sacred waters that had been collected from around the world and asked her to use those vibrations to help her heal the condition of the sea. I dowsed afterward and the lines were completely gone! The condition at that time was so desperate that not only birds and fish were dying, but people as well. Thousands of dead fish littered the shore of the sea. The water was deep brown from the sewage, and it was so foul that you could smell the septic stench from a town ten miles away.

Clean up the Salton Sea

The deva there told us "not to worry, come back in a couple of weeks." To my mind, it seemed impossible for there to be any improvement in this dire situation in just a couple of weeks. We were too busy to come back then and returned instead in March. What we saw was amazing. The sea had no odor at all, there were no dead fish, and the water was so clear you could see the rocks at the bottom. We also saw a number of birds at a time when they were supposed to be migrating north. Since that time this miraculous improvement has made the Los Angeles, San Diego, and Salton Sea papers a number of times, each time stunning and mystifying the scientists, who cannot explain the unexpected turn of events. All of that from just a thirty-minute process on our parts. What rejuvenating powers nature holds!

When we asked the local people if there had been any action taken to clean up the Salton Sea, we learned that a major multimillion dollar project was stuck in legislation and had not even been passed yet, so no outer action had been taken in the two months since we'd been there last. A couple of months later a friend returned from camping in the area and described it as "pristine." This was difficult to believe, but when I flew over the sea by plane a week later, I saw for myself that the water was indeed blue and that there was no smog or pollution anywhere.

Potential for Healing Oceans

An interesting phenomenon is the occurrence of whales and dolphins in areas where work is being done with the Harmonizers. In three different locations—Seattle, Los Angeles, and Cape Cod—whales and dolphins appeared in the bay and harbors where they had never been sighted before. They appeared to be attracted to the energy of the Harmonizers and the clearing frequencies being broadcast. In one instance off the coast of British Columbia during a whale-watching trip, all ninety-seven Orca whales who live in the area surrounded our boat. They had reversed their northerly direction up the coast to come down to where we were and, according to the boat captain, were moving at a record speed to meet us. All three resident pods of Orcas had encircled our little boat, when one of the whales came directly toward us and went beneath it. According to the person in our boat who had the ability to communicate with whales, this whale was the leader of the pod and was taking the frequencies of our Harmonizer and tapes back to the rest of the pod to broadcast throughout the waters they patrol. If the whales are able to take these frequencies and broadcast them throughout the oceans, the implications are vast. It means there is potential for a complete healing of our oceans.

Christan Hummel travels around the world to set up environmental clearing networks in local areas. For more information, visit www.earthtransitions.com.

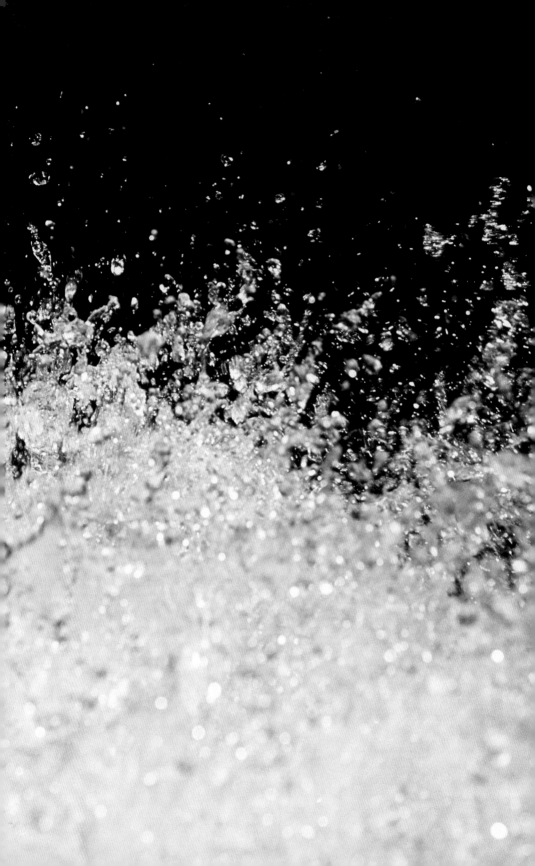

6

Revitalizing Your Own Water

What You Need to Know

A NUMBER OF READERS may be having difficulty putting together all the technical data presented in the preceding chapters. Therefore, this chapter provides a summary of the characteristics of water and the procedures or techniques that have been introduced for its activation and revitalization.

1. As water is a highly sensitive substance, it reacts immediately to outside influences, both positively and negatively. These reactions include its ability to restructure itself on a molecular level, an increase or reduction of its vitality (photon emission), and its memory, depending on how it is imprinted or revitalized.

2. Healthy, vital water is able to process impurities, pollutants, and stress—in other words, it has the ability to regenerate. This regeneration is connected to its swirling movement, its natural spiral coiling (implosion). Similarly, it has the ability to assimilate negative information—at least up to a certain point.

3. When polluted water is put in contact with a spring or another form of concentrated vital energy (chi, orgone, tachyons, and so

on) that is harmoniously structured on the subatomic level, not only will it revitalize but it will also recover its innate power to purify and heal, by virtue of the biocatalytic process. (See the two photos on page 26 illustrating the Hagalis method for the dynamization of water.)

4. Many procedures and techniques have been developed over the past several decades for producing concentrated forms of bioenergy and transmitting it to devitalized—dirty or polluted—water.

5. Revitalized water that has been redynamized on the molecular level recovers its innate ability to absorb oxygen and loses surface tension. It therefore becomes softer and more fluid. The minerals that remain suspended in such water and make it hard are carried away in the water instead of being deposited on the walls of blood vessels or water pipes.

Furthermore, biologically healthy water:

➤ More easily rids itself of impurities (meaning fewer cleaning products are needed).

➤ Is better at eliminating wastes from the human body.

➤ Is a better bonding agent in production of cement, paint, and so forth.

➤ More readily absorbs oxygen, nutritive substances, and minerals.

➤ Encourages the germination of plants.

➤ Helps to preserve cut flowers, and fresh fruits and vegetables.

➤ Is a superior conductor of heat (thus reducing the energy needed in water-based heating systems).

Dynamized, or revitalized, water is an important factor in the health and vitality of the living entities it nurtures, whether they are human beings, animals, or plants. It contributes to the harmony of biological processes. For example, if we subject a water sample to revolutions of the right (clockwise) in a dynamization procedure or technique, it rebalances itself on the subatomic level. Pathogenic substances shrink or vanish and the immune system is strengthened in the person consuming this water.

TECHNIQUES FOR BIOENERGETIC DYNAMIZATION OF WATER

It is impossible to introduce in one book all the procedures and techniques currently commercially available for water dynamization. Those who wish to learn more can consult the resources section (see page 13) or search on the Internet. Although many of the websites are in German, nearly all offer English translation.

There are new discoveries all the time, but for readers wishing to purchase a device, this summary describes the current predominant techniques for dynamization of water.

1. *Filtering through mechanical methods.* In any water dynamization device equipped with a filter, this process almost always takes place through reverse osmosis or active charcoal. Active charcoal will not filter out minerals (iron, potassium, magnesium, and so on), nitrites, nitrates, or pollution residue; but reverse osmosis will rid the water of these substances, as it only allows water molecules to pass through. (See also "Types of Water Filters" in chapter 5, page 97.)

2. *Permanent magnets.* The primary advantage of magnets is that they alter the structure of the ions of calcium and magnesium suspended in water so thoroughly that lime scaling does not occur in the plumbing or collect on the walls of blood vessels when the water is consumed. Simultaneously, magnets imprint a whirling movement on the water, which breaks up the undesirable molecular clusters, erases their "memory," and improves the reactivity of the water. The water recovers its original vitality and is able to capture and dispense new information.

3. *Water turbulence (the implosion system developed by Viktor Schauberger).* Through a special fitting, clockwise spirals imprint a swirling action on dirty or polluted water. This movement deconstructs the molecular clusters caused by pollution and erases the negative, pathogenic information that has collected there. Spiral movements produce bioenergy, which catalyzes the regeneration of

the water. The water is once again able to absorb oxygen in sufficient quantity, thereby regaining its ability to purify itself.

4. *Dynamization of water through concentrated natural energy (bioenergy, orgone, and tachyons).* Here the vitalization of the water takes place on the subatomic level. The emission of photons is visibly intensified by this method, and water that has been treated in this way can once again remember its original structure. Information linked to pollutants is erased, and the water's spin is rebalanced. Water recovers all of its vitality and robustness and can therefore better resist attacks from bacteria or pollutants (this is the case with water at Lourdes and the Ganges River). This water dynamization process intensifies the regenerative abilities of devitalized water as well as its biocatalytic power.

5. *Passing water over semiprecious or mountain stones.* This completely natural procedure activates and vitalizes dirty or polluted water on the bioenergetic level and also transforms "juvenile" water into more mature forms (for example, water coming from artesian wells). Water that has been treated this way becomes permeated by the vibrations of the stones and adopts their molecular structure. It becomes better tasting and can be consumed without any adverse consequences.

6. *Transfer of primal information.* Here the polluted water or wastewater is put in either direct or indirect contact with geometric shapes, a very pure water spring, crystals, or even a water of light. The polluted water can be permeated by the inherent qualities of the information-carrying water and reorganize itself on the molecular level.

7. *Imprinting of micro-information.* Injecting wastewater or polluted water with beneficial vibrational frequencies that have been explicitly determined will bring life back to this kind of water. For example, infusing a lake or an aquarium with information concerning oxygen teaches this water to spontaneously supply itself with oxygen and thereby improve its ability to neutralize the harmful and pathogenic effects of pollutants. This procedure, as

we saw earlier, is effective for decontaminating fairly large bodies of water, even those that have been heavily polluted.

Some water dynamization devices are equipped with programs that allow the user to modulate the remedial frequency mandated by the distinctive characteristics of the water to be treated.

8. *Carrier/support material.* The efficiency of a water dynamization device depends upon, among other things, the carrier material used for information transfer.

If the information carrier is water, the device in question runs the risk of losing much of its effectiveness over time. Furthermore, given water's high degree of resonance, the water is at risk of capturing vibrations emanating from either the surrounding environment or the water itself, which then have the potential of influencing the water in their proximity.

Water as a support material can be stabilized with salt. Saline water stabilizes the information that has been transmitted, making it less quickly erased.

Crystals, green clay, and certain mineral powders are durable and have specific features that make them excellent carrier material for information for water.

Not all water dynamization devices utilize carrier materials. For some the dynamization is generated by internal activity; their vibrations are generated by geometric models. The function and durability of such devices are practically unlimited.

9. *Radionics.* The possibilities offered by this technique for activating and revitalizing water are staggering, but it belongs only in the hands of professionals with specific knowledge, integrity, and consciousness.

SHOULD TAP WATER BE FILTERED?

This question arises regarding the different procedures or techniques for the bioenergetic dynamization of water that have been presented here. Just how much of the polluting substances do they actually eliminate? Or, if not eliminate, how greatly do they reduce the toxicity of these substances?

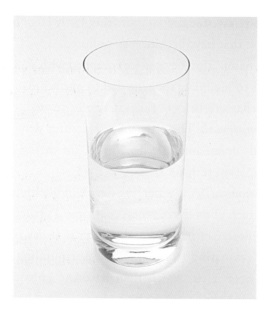

The purity of our tap water is far from guaranteed.

These substances can include heavy metals, pesticides, asbestos fibers, pharmaceutical residues, and so forth.

Our tap water is far from free of pollutants. Public authorities set maximum rates and then give the local water boards responsibility for monitoring water quality to ensure that these thresholds are not exceeded. Because these rates are set in accordance with the criteria of the economy, politics, and procedural realities, the purity of our tap water is far from guaranteed. In both Germany and the United States, for example, the maximum rate of aluminum in tap water is currently 0.2 mg per liter. Since aluminum is suspected to be a factor in neurological dysfunction and a range of other illnesses, this figure is high enough to elicit dismay from most physicians and health practitioners.

Truthfully speaking, a certain number of pollutants are quite simply absent from the lists drawn up by public works departments and thus are not subject to any monitoring or control. Among these pollutants are hormonal residues from factory farming, which eventually will infiltrate our water tables in the same way that improperly discarded prescription drugs already have. Can the biotechnical procedures for activating and revitalizing water eliminate the hazards of this kind of pollutant? If not, it would make sense to include a filter that would address this need.

Bioenergetic Processes Used in Purifying Water

Before addressing the possibility of additional filtration for our water, I am going to briefly revisit the various bioenergetic techniques available for dissolving both pollutants and the water's memory of these pollutants.

Swirling Movements

Because the swirling clockwise movement that these methods imprint upon the water is quite powerful, it flattens and breaks apart the undesirable molecular clusters. The water then loses its chaotic structure, and pollutants and impurities are broken down into their constituent elements (at least with respect to organic substances). This stage of the treatment vitalizes the water.

Magnetic Micro-whirlpools

This dynamization procedure causes effects quite similar to the swirling movement method described above but uses magnetic impulses to break apart the unwanted molecular clusters.

Polarity Reversal

As we saw earlier, the principal characteristic of polluted or devitalized water is the direction of its rotations (to the left, or counterclockwise, rather than to the right), which is a reverse spin on the atomic and subatomic levels. This imbalance not only leeches the water of its energy but also arranges the pollutants into fixed positions. Bioenergetic techniques can reverse this polarity.

Once the reversal by the informing polarity has been achieved, the water treated in this way will be characterized by at least a balanced spin, if not by primarily clockwise rotations. A water of this nature no longer offers any footholds for pollutants, and germs and bacteria are unable to proliferate; in human terms, the immune system has been restored. It is because of its balanced and stable spin that the water from Lourdes or the Ganges River does not pass on to others the viruses or bacteria from the ill people who bathe there. Pollutants and poisons are prevented from spreading in waters like this, which are known as holy or sacred waters; instead, they are gradually confined to a solitary existence. Eventually any organic substances will decompose and break apart into their basic constituent elements.

⌒

These three modalities of biophysical water dynamization are known to be highly effective and far superior to biochemical procedures. This has been verified repeatedly. Most water dynamization devices combine two procedures in one device. Given the fact that water pollution has become increasingly complex and stubbornly resistant to dissolution (especially the pollution caused by pharmaceutical wastes), combined use is strongly recommended.

Dissolution of Chemical Substances and Heavy Metals

Another question that often comes up is whether the bioenergetic revitalization processes can dissolve chemical substances such as chlorine, metals such as aluminum, and heavy metals such as lead. A priori, this seems highly unlikely.

In bodies of open water—lakes, ponds, pools, and so on—it can be assumed that pollutants are absorbed by all kinds of small creatures or tiny fish. But in closed systems of water distribution, such as tap water or coolant, how is it possible to explain why, several weeks after the installation of a bioenergetic dynamization device, dirty water from heating ducts, laden with all kinds of impurities, has become crystal clear once more? Where did the rust, the traces of lead, and the traces of copper go? Did they simply evaporate as if by magic? The answer is yes.

The disappearance of these traces of pollution is mysterious not only to biochemists but also to the inventors of these water dynamization devices. Do black holes also exist in the microcosm? Can they swallow matter, just as their larger counterparts in the macrocosm do? We don't yet know. Could one consequence of the bioenergetic activation and revitalization of wastewater be the production of microorganisms that feed on pollutants and transform them?

The absorption of pollutants by tiny living organisms is a well-known phenomena. This is why so many are now commonly using microorganisms—with most satisfying results, by the way—for cleaning garbage dumps and other areas polluted by chemical materials. Microorganisms could almost be

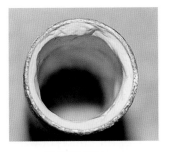

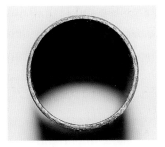

A heating pipe with heavy calcium deposits

The same pipe just a few weeks after the installation of a water dynamization device (hardly a trace of mineral sedimentation)

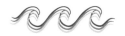

described as the alchemists of pollution. Could an analogous phenomenon be taking place with the dynamization of wastewater and polluted water? We are still a long way from knowing all the answers.

Some manufacturers advise customers to integrate an additional filter into their water dynamization system, either an active charcoal filter or one that works using reverse osmosis. This is a very sensible approach. I say this because water dynamization procedures excel at ridding tap water of most pollutants, but they cannot remove possible traces of arsenic, for example, which has been found in the public water systems of nearly half of the United States.

GENERAL GUIDELINES FOR REVITALIZING YOUR OWN WATER

I would advise all those who wish to seriously explore activating and revitalizing their water supply to begin at the beginning. What I mean by this is to *sharpen your sensitivity* to the element water. This involves learning to observe and taste water. I would like to offer some general suggestions.

➤ Avoid drinking water in a mechanical, unconscious fashion. Instead, take small sips while feeling fully present in the action: feel the taste of the water on your tongue in the same way a wine taster tastes wine. Next, concentrate on feeling the refreshing and revitalizing effect the water has on your body.

➤ When preparing tea with ordinary water, observe the color of that water and the traces it leaves. This will help you learn how to tell the difference between a devitalized water and a dynamized water.

➤ When bathing, whether in a bathtub, a swimming pool, or the ocean, really experience the feel of the water on your skin. But even more importantly, take stock of the effects of water on your body afterward. You will realize that this sensation is varied, depending upon the quality of the water.

One of the most basic ways of dynamizing water, a way that is as old as it is effective, is to *thank and bless* it, but this only works if you truly put your heart into it. There are those of us who associate acts like this to out-dated religious beliefs. They have a right to their opinions, but we should nonetheless recall that benediction and expression of gratitude have concrete effects on water—effects that have been verified scientifically. For example, we can refer to the photos taken by Masaru Emoto that demonstrate that the morphology of a glass of water was altered by simply writing "Thank you" on a piece of paper and taping it to the side of the glass. The structure of the water crystals became more complex and more harmonious.

Once you have developed a certain degree of sensitivity to water, you may choose to dynamize water with crystals. The instructions for doing this are provided in chapter 5 in the section entitled "Revitalizing Water with Crystals" (page 102).

When it comes to products for activating and revitalizing water, rather than buy an expensive device right away, you may prefer to start with something small and moderately priced, such as the products offered by the Alvito Company (see the section entitled "Alvito: A Solution for All Your Water Problems," page 92). There are also the products offered by the American David Wagner (see the section entitled "Water Vitalized by Tachyons," page 97). (Also see the resources section of this book.)

To see for yourself the difference revitalized water can make, you may want to purchase bottled dynamized water (water of light, levitated water, Grander water, water treated by tachyons, and so forth) and perform the

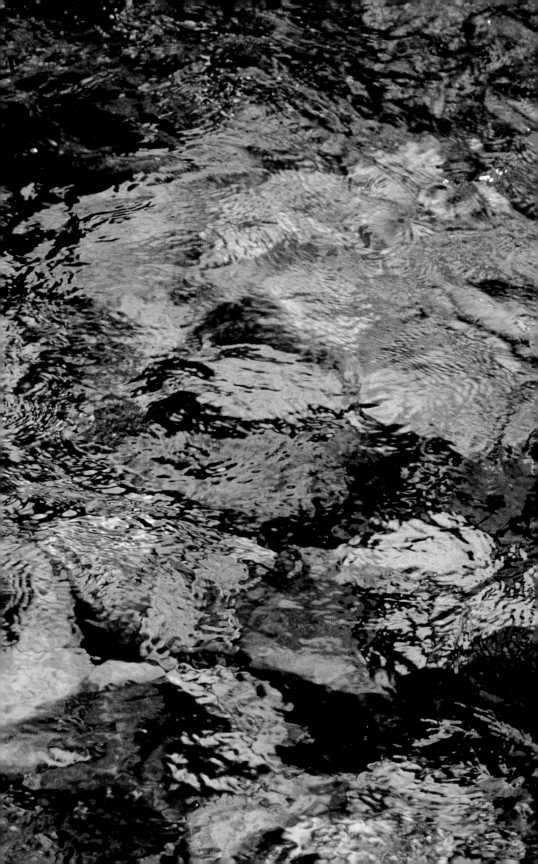

following experiment: Arrange flowers in two different vases. Use ordinary tap water for one, but add several drops of dynamized water to the other. Observe them every day and see what happens.

Following are several common sense recommendations for water preservation.

- ➤ Dynamized water should be kept out of direct sunlight in a cool location. The molecules in lukewarm water have a tendency to become less complex and harmonious.
- ➤ Keep the water in glass or ceramic containers—avoid plastic containers like the plague!
- ➤ Metal will preserve the cool temperature of water for the longest time. On the other hand, it has the disadvantage of attracting static electricity, and this will be passed into the water. You should also avoid placing a metal thermos near a computer.

There Is No Ideal Device, Only Solutions Adapted to Specific Needs

Water dynamization techniques are based on a certain number of parameters: the nature of the support material, the combination of the different components of that support material, the initial water quality, and the hardness of the water to be treated. Analyses of the same water, even when performed by the same laboratory, rarely provide identical results. We need to remember that water is a living substance that is ceaselessly moving and changing, and these fluctuations will always be reflected. Water also reacts quite strongly to the moon and the planets. This is why many people feel their nerves are on edge during a full moon. It is due to the specific quality of the water molecules in their bodies.

We should also recall that there is no single ideal device for reactivating and revitalizing water—one that can be adapted to any need. This is why every dynamization device is conditioned at purchase to best respond to its intended use. This holds true for individual consumers as well as businesses and towns. The manufacturer should specify the amount of water a device can treat, the modalities of installation, and its cost. And why not perform kinesiology tests as well? Obviously the dynamized water needs of a family living in Paris will be different from those of a business in Albuquerque.

Device Guarantees

While most of these European-based companies guarantee their devices for periods of years, they cannot guarantee their effectiveness. By scientific standards their effectiveness, even though results have been verified, is attributable to blind faith or a placebo effect. Current legislation does not take the subtle planes into account!

Personally, I recommend that any buyer of a device for revitalizing water get a written guarantee from the vendor that he will be allowed to return the device in the event it does not keep its promises. Verification procedures do exist. For example we have the Hagalis method and electroluminescence (biophotonics), among others. The serious companies will generally raise no objections to this request.

Basic Recommendations for Installing a Water Dynamization Device

To close, I would like to offer some very concrete recommendations about what to do before buying and installing one of these systems or devices.

- ❥ Make sure that any underground cable bringing electricity into the house is not running next to a water pipe. If it is, the water is at risk of becoming contaminated by electromagnetic pollution, which would reduce the effectiveness of any device for dynamizing water. If this is the case, consult an expert who can fix the situation.
- ❥ Avoid installing a water dynamization system or device above a subterranean water vein or in proximity to a vein of underground water. Here, too, there is a risk of contamination by undesirable vibrations. If possible, consult a water dowser who can advise you on how to cancel out the negative effects.
- ❥ Relay antennas reduce the effects of water dynamization devices. The electromagnetic waves (with a reverse spin) they generate have the vexing propensity of clinging to the sheathing of

specially magnetized steel. If you live in the proximity of an antenna like this, ask the manufacturers of the water dynamization device you are contemplating buying if they can work out protective measures for your specific situation.

〜 A water dynamization device may initially slough off large amounts of calcification and rust into the pipes; this period lasts from two to eight weeks in most cases. If the device does not include a filtration step capable of removing these products, then it is better not to drink the tap water until the water has settled down.

〜 Integration of water dynamization devices into water meters may not be permitted.

〜 Apartment dwellers should place their water dynamization device on the pipe carrying water into their apartment, most often found in the bathroom. They may be able to install a special filter beneath or on the kitchen sink.

As you can see, it is not very difficult to revitalize your daily water. And the benefits are well worth it; you will very soon recover your appetite for this vital resource that is so essential to health and well-being.

"Good Morning," said the little prince.

"Good morning," said the salesclerk. This was a salesclerk who sold pills invented to quench thirst. Swallow one a week and you no longer feel any need to drink.

"Why do you sell these pills?"

"They save so much time," the salesclerk said. "Experts have calculated that you can save fifty-three minutes a week."

"And what do you do with those fifty-three minutes?"

"Whatever you like."

"If I had fifty-three minutes to spend as I liked," the little prince said to himself, "I'd walk very slowly toward a water fountain . . ."

Antoine de Saint-Exupéry, *Le Petit Prince,*
translated by Richard Howard

Resources

There are hundreds of websites and companies worldwide that now provide devices similar to those described in this book. The list below is merely a representative sample. Most of the European websites offer pages in English.

USA AND CANADA

Cocoon Nutrition
274 East Hamilton Avenue, Suite G
Campbell, CA 95008
Tel: (888) 988-3325
www.cocoonnutrition.org

For information about David Wagner and his tachyonized products, go to
www.planet-tachyon.com

EMR Labs, LLC
P.O. Box 33
Cascade, CO 80809-0033
Tel: (800) 435-1392
www.quantumbalancing.com
www.biophotonanalyzer.com

The Schauberger-inspired line of Wellness water products
is available at
www.amazon.com

Unitative Productions, Inc.
1794 SE 22nd Avenue
Portland, OR 97214
Tel: (503) 284-1658
Fax: (815) 301-8182
www.tachyon-energy-products.com

Water Tubes Water Vortex Systems
P.O. Box 1295
Bandera, TX 78003
Tel: (830) 796-8377
www.vortexwatersystems.com

World Living Water Systems
432 North Dollarton Hwy.
North Vancouver, BC V7G 1N1
Canada
Tel: (604) 990-5462
Fax: (604) 904-7455
www.alivewater.net

U.K. AND EUROPE

Alvito GmbH
Hillerstraße 25
90429 Nürnberg, Germany
Tel: 09 11 321 521
Fax: 09 11 321 5222
e-mail: info@alvito.de
www.alvito.de

Aguavital
C.Balandro 13.2.D
E-28042 Madrid, Spain
Tel: 91 320 60 59
www.aguavitalymas.com

BIOTAC Consulting
Tachyon Technology
Champ Belluet 18
CH—1807 Blonay, Switzerland
Tel: 41 21 943 3874
Fax: 41 21 943 3873
www.biotac.ch

Centre for Implosion Research
P.O. Box 38
Plymouth PL7 5YX, U.K.
Tel: 44 17 52 345 552
Fax: 44 17 52 338 569
www.implosionresearch.com

Clean-Water
Lavoigne Madsen ApS
Egholmvej 8–10
DK 7160 Toerring, Denmark
Tel: 45 76 902 410
Fax: 45 76 902 419
www.clean-water.dk

Elisa Energiesysteme
Lampertsham 7
D-83349 Palling, Germany
Tel: 49 08 629 1819
Fax: 49 08 629 1885
e-mail: info@elisaenergiesysteme.com
www.waterresearch.biz/index.html

Feng Shui for Health
Ambermill Farm, Oakerthorpe
Alfreton DE55 7LL, U.K.
Tel: 44 17 73 833 228

GranderWasser
Bergwerksweg 10
6373 Jochberg, Austria
Tel: 43 53 55 5615
Fax: 43 55 53 5459
e-mail: info@wasser.at
www.granderwasser.com
http://usa.grander.biz

Pythagoras Kepler System
Kaltenbach 162
4821 Lauffen, Bad Ischl, Austria
www.oks.or.at

Roland Plocher integral-technik
Torenstrasse 8
D–88709 Meersburg, Germany
Tel: 49 75 32 43 330
Fax: 49 75 32 43 3310
www.plocher.de/englisch

AUSTRALIA
AND SOUTH AFRICA

Ankh de Haan
P.O. Box 85
Woy Woy, NSW 2256
Australia
Tel: 61 413 696 816
e-mail: info@crystalquarters.net
www.crystalquarters.net

Mary Martin
Orionis CC
P.O. Box 11226, Rynfield 1514
South Africa
Tel: 27 11 849 8088
Fax: 27 11 849 3838
e-mail: mary_n@telkomsa.net

Westgate Distributors CC
94 Townsend Street
Goodwood 7460
South Africa
Tel/Fax: 27 21 592 3366
e-mail: westgate@gem.co.za

SOUTH AMERICA

Soal Vidas, A.C.
Calle Los Zorzales
130 of 60
San Isidro, Lima
Peru
e-mail: info@soalvida.com
www.soalvida.com

Bioenergia EIRL
Lo Beltran 1946
7640558 Vitacura
Santiago
Chile

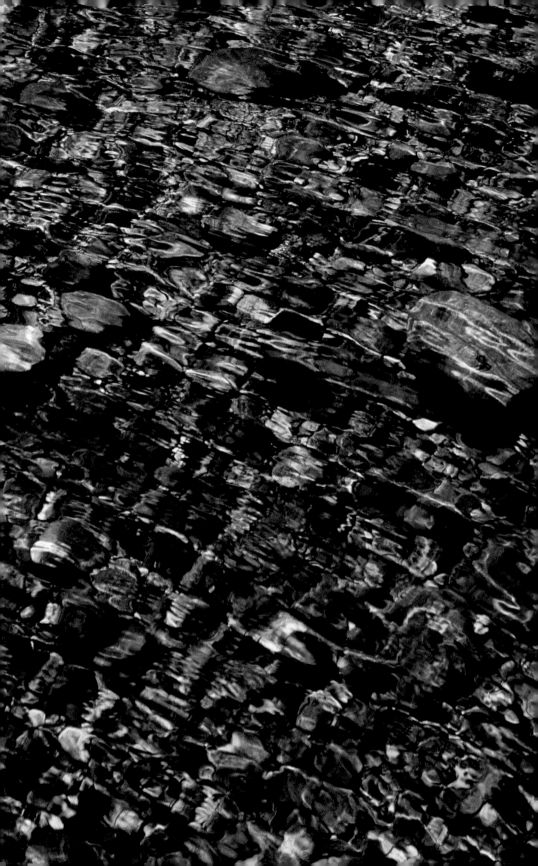

Recommended
Reading and Listening

The following books and audio recordings—about water, or inspired by water—
are recommended by the author.

BOOKS

Alexandersson, Olaf. *Living Water: Viktor Schauberger and the Secrets of Natural Energy,* 2nd ed. N.p.: Newleaf, 2002.

Batmanghelidji, Faridun. *Your Body's Many Cries for Water.* Vienna, Va.: Global Health Solutions, 1995.

Bischof, Marco. *Tachyonen, Orgonenergie, Skalarwellen: Feinstoffliche Felder zwischen Mythos und Wissenschaft.* Baden, Switz.: AT Verlag, 2002.

Braun, Ernest F. *Wasserkristalle: Zauberwelt auf gefrorenen Wassertropfen.* Baden, Switz.: AT Verlag, 2004.

Coats, Callum. *Living Energies: An Exposition of Concepts Related to the Theories of Viktor Schauberger.* Bath, U.K.: Gateway Books, 2002.

Davidson, John. *The Secret of the Creative Vacuum: Man and the Energy Dance.* London: C. W. Daniel Company/Random House, 2004.

———. *Subtle Energy.* London: C. W. Daniel Company/Random House, 2004.

Dalla Via, Gudrun. *Les eaux d'énergie et de lumière: Le pouvoir guérisseur de l'eau des sanctuaires sacrés.* Paris: Éditions Véga, 2006.

Emoto, Masaru. *The Hidden Messages in Water.* New York: Atria, 2005.

———. *The True Power of Water: Healing and Discovering Ourselves.* New York: Atria, 2005.

———. *The Healing Power of Water.* Carlsbad, Calif.: Hay House, 2007.

Hacheney, Friedrich. *Levitiertes Wasser in Forschung und Anwendung.* Andechs, Ger.: Dingfelder Verlag, 1994.

Hacheney, Wilfried. *Wasser: Wesen zweier Welten.* Peiting, Ger.: Michaels-Verlag, 2003.

Hendel, Barbara. *Wasser vom Reinsten: So optimieren Sie Ihr Leitungswasser.* Herrsching, Ger.: INA Verlag, 2002.

———. *Water and Salt: The Essence of Life.* New York: Natural Resources, Inc., 2003.

Lautewasser, Alexander. *Images sonores de l'eau.* Paris: Editions Médicis, 2005.

Kronberger, Hans, and Siegbert Lattacher. *Auf der Spur des Wasserrätsels: Von Viktor Schauberger bis Johann Grander.* Vienna: Uranus Verlag, 2000.

Manning, Jeanne. *Energie: Bessere Alternativen für eine saubere Welt.* Aachen, Ger.: Omega Verlag, 2002.

Optiz, Christian. *Unbegrenzte Lebenskraft durch Tachyonen: Der neue Weg zu körperlicher Heilung und geistiger Entwicklung.* Fribourg im Brisgau, Ger.: Hans-Nietsch Verlag, 1997.

Reich, Wilhelm. *Selected Writings: An Introduction to Orgonomy.* New York: Farrar, Strauss, Giroux, 1963.

Schauberger, Viktor. *Viktor the Water Wizard: The Extraordinary Powers of Natural Water.* Bath, U.K.: Gateway, 1998.

Schwenk, Theodor. *Sensitive Chaos: The Creation of Flowing Forms in Water and Air.* East Sussex, U.K.: Rudolf Steiner Press, 2004.

Selbmann, Sibylle. *Mythos Wasser: Symbolik und Kulturgeschichte.* Karlsruhe, Ger.: Badenia Verlag, 1995.

Senf, Bernd. *Die Wiederentdeckung des Lebendigen: Erforschung der Lebensenergie durch Reich, Schauberger, Lakhovsky u.a.* Aachen, Ger.: Omega Verlag, 2003.

Sheldrake, Rupert. *Presence of the Past.* Rochester, Vt.: Inner Traditions, 1995.

———. *A New Science of Life*, revised and expanded. Rochester, Vt.: Inner Traditions, 2009.

———. *Rebirth of Nature.* Rochester, Vt.: Inner Traditions, 1994.

———. *Seven Experiments that Can Change the World.* Rochester, Vt.: Inner Traditions, 2002.

Wexler, Richard, Wolfgang Hauer, contrib. *Garten und Schwimmteiche: Bau— Bepflanzung—Pflege.* Graz, Austria: L. Stocker Verlag, 1998.

MUSIC

Deuter. *Sea and Silence.* Santa Fe, N. Mex: New Earth Records, 2002.

Dury, Laurent. *Mer de la sérénité.* Paris: Origins, 2000.

Handel, Georg Friedrich. *Water Music.* John Eliot Gardiner, conductor. N.p.: Philips, 2001.

Kamal. *Reiki Whale Song.* Santa Fe, N. Mex: New Earth Records, 2001.

Khalid, Bodhi. *Mother Earth Carry Me.* N.p.: Silenzio, 2005

Niggli and Simona. *L'Écho des rivages 3.* Paris: Origins, 1998, 2007.

Prem, Joshua. *Water down Ganga.* Santa Fe, N. Mex: New Earth Records, 2003.

Samaya. *Water Spirit.* Burgrain, Ger.: Koha Verlag, 2002.

Samudra. *La Voix de l'océan.* Paris: Origins, 2004.

Smetana, Bedrich. *Die Moldau.* Herbert von Karajan, conductor. Hamburg, Ger.: Deutsche Grammophon, 1995.

Stacke, Ivan. *Rivages et ressacs.* Paris: Origins, 1999.

Various Artists. *Spa Lounge.* Santa Fe, N. Mex: New Earth Records, 2003.

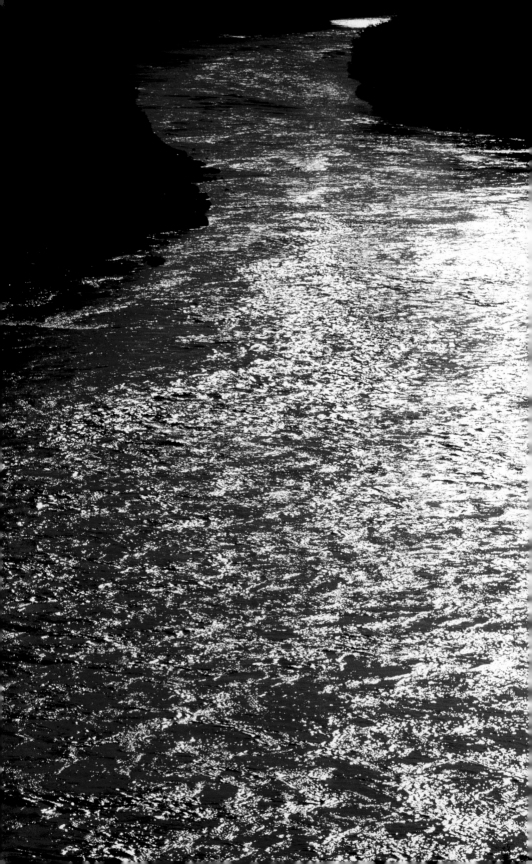

Illustration Credits

page 6 (top). Hans-Dietrich Korth, Aeroclub Tauberbischofsheim e.V., 2002.

page 11. A. Pichler, Kitzbühel.

page 26. Hagalis AG, Aftholderberg.

page 29. Labor P. Wandfluh, Elisa Energiesysteme archives, Lampertsham.

page 43. Institut für aquatische Wasserarbeit, Freiburg.

page 46. Drawing by Birgit Pfeifer, Sottrum.

page 53. J. Fischer, Bad Fallingbostel.

pages 76, 86, 87, 89, 91. Weber Bio-Energie-Systeme, Zierenberg.

page 95. Alvito GmbH, Nuremberg.

page 100. Antares Design, Frickenhausen.

pages 104, 106. Vielharmonie GmbH, Sulzberg.

page 107. A. Pichler, Kitzbühel.

page 109. Elisa Energiesysteme, Lampertsham.

pages 113, 133. Weber Bio-Energie-Systeme, Zierenberg.

Index

Page numbers in *italics* refer to figures.